THE

ONE MINUTE
WORKOUT

THE

ONE MINUTE
WORKOUT

Build Fat-Burning Lean Muscle,
Massive Strength, and Better Health
in Just 60 Seconds a Day!

Raymond Wu, M.D.

E2 Press books are available at special discounts for bulk purchase. Special editions or book excerpts can also be created to specification. For details, contact the E2 Press Special Sales Manager at sales@E2-Press.com.

www.OneMinWorkout.com

Publisher's Cataloging-In-Publication Data
(Prepared by The Donohue Group, Inc.)

Wu, Raymond.
  The one minute workout : build fat-burning lean muscle, massive strength, and better health in just 60 seconds a day! / Raymond Wu, M.D. -- First edition.

    pages : illustrations ; cm

  Includes bibliographical references.
  ISBN-13: 978-1-941388-00-6
  ISBN-10: 1-941388-00-0

  1. Exercise. 2. Muscle strength. 3. Physical fitness. I. Title.

RA781 .W8 2014
613.7/1   2014944284

This book is dedicated to each person who has ever wanted or tried to get in shape. Exercise not for the sake of it, but to empower and enable you to get more out of life.

Acknowledgments

Without a wealth of experiences to draw from, the idea for the One Minute Workout would never have come to fruition. In particular, my teachers, coaches, instructors, and patients have imparted me with invaluable knowledge and skills over the years. To all of you, I thank you from the bottom of my heart.

Like a seed, an idea requires support and nourishment to sprout and flourish. To this end, I would like to thank my wife, Cathy, for her unwavering support over the years. You have helped me in countless ways and shaped this into what it is today. I would also like to thank my parents, my brother, his wife, and my wife's parents for their support throughout this lengthy endeavor. Thanks to Dr. Stanley Tsao for his help since the beginning of this project. I deeply appreciate your instrumental analysis, assistance with content preparation, and most importantly, your steadfast friendship through the ups and downs.

To my good friends Tony Marquez and Amber Kuo, thank you for your support and advice over the years, and for providing your facilities at EKF Martial Arts in Chicago, IL for shooting the photography in this book. Thanks to Wesley Chu for his guidance on writing and publishing. In addition, I'd like to thank Alexandra Kollontai for her expert editing assistance.

Feedback is the instrument that sculpts effectiveness out of raw ideas. I would like to thank all of my beta-readers and testers for their time and priceless feedback. I would especially like to thank the following: John Wamser, Taylor Choi-Marquez, Seul Oh, Wayne Wu, Dr. Todd Occomy, Peggy Chung, Mike Palmer, Nick Hennigan, Daniel Schwab, Natalie Minh, Stephanie Minster, Duane Mangahas, Rod Stevens, Dr. Michael Fang, Elizabeth McManus, Dr. Michael Cho, Pius Wong, and Jason Moy. Thank you for joining me in this journey to improve the life of others.

聚沙成塔、持之以恒

Just as sand can be gathered to build giant towers,
small but persistent efforts can achieve anything.
—Chinese Proverb

Contents

Section V: Advanced Progressions & Exercises

Appendix

A Word from the Author

Thud … Thud! What was that? I try to look around, but it is pitch black. *CLANG! THUD!* The sounds get louder as I slowly come to my senses. I open my eyes groggily, squinting at my surroundings through the fluorescent lights. The haze over my consciousness dissolves, and I sheepishly realize that I had fallen asleep at the gym … again. Still exhausted and depleted from a 30-hour shift at the hospital, I am too tired to work out at all. As I head to the locker room to change, I tell myself, "So much for getting back in shape … at least I got to the gym." Driving home, I can't help but think that there has to be a better and easier way to get in shape. A few years later, I have the answer.

From Fit to Fat, and Back Again

The One Minute Workout system was born from my own personal struggle to take care of my body during a particularly difficult time in my life. I used to be very active and in great shape. Like a lot of young people, if I wasn't in the gym lifting weights, I was playing a sport or training for an event. My resting pulse rate was under 40, and like most people in their 20s, I felt invincible. Not exercising never crossed my mind.

Unfortunately, this all started to change when I began my first job after medical school. As a resident physician, I often worked 60+ hour weeks, which included 24-to-30-hour-long shifts at a time. The long irregular hours left me with little time and energy to exercise.

As a doctor in the age of electronic medical records, I spent most of my working day sitting down. If I wasn't sitting down and seeing patients, I was either at the computer reviewing lab data and writing progress notes on patients, or on the phone coordinating care with other doctors. After work, I spent several more hours sitting, either studying or at the computer. With little time to cook, frozen pizzas and fast food were my go-to dinners. When I was lucky enough to find some spare time, I would try to go to the Kung Fu school where I used to train during medical school. However, I often found myself nodding off from lack of sleep before classes even started! Needless to say, I had a very sedentary and unhealthy lifestyle, which was exactly what I counseled my patients to avoid.

The consequences of this unhealthy lifestyle crept up on me as silently as a ninja. First, I started having back and leg pain whenever I sat down. I could never find a comfortable position to sit in for more than few minutes. Next, I noticed that it was getting harder to bend over or squat down. Simple things like leaning over to tie my shoe laces seemed to take more effort. It felt like my belly kept getting in the way, although it didn't look any bigger in the mirror. So, I chalked it up to the food still in my belly from the previous meal. Finally, I started finding it difficult to play the sports I loved. My mid-section kept getting in the way every time I tried to bend my body, whether to dodge a kick or to lunge after a ball. But again, I waved away the warning signs, because when I looked in the mirror, I didn't look *that* much different than before.

Looking back, the reason for these changes was obvious. Despite being a doctor and having seen plenty of overweight patients, I didn't realize at the time that I was getting fat on the inside. This fat was accumulating in my abdomen, "hiding" between the organs so that it was not visible. All that fat was making it difficult to move around like I used to. Yet from the outside, there wasn't much evidence of its presence. Although not quite as flat or firm as they used to be, my six-pack abs were still very much intact. And this was why I was still in denial.

A few years later, I finished my medical residency, but it was too late. The inevitable had already happened. The six-pack had vanished, replaced by a "one-pack," or possibly a "two-pack" if I flexed really hard and the lighting was just right. The once-defined muscles in my arms and legs had become shapeless, and I had gained more weight than I cared to admit. I kept telling myself that I would get back in shape, but the demands of life always got the better of me. One day, my mom exclaimed "You've gotten fat!" That was my wakeup call.

Those were words that I never expected to hear, and it snapped me out of denial. Even though I have always hated cardio training, I started running. When it was too cold outside, I tried using the treadmill, but that quickly became boring. I also went to the gym whenever I could to lift weights, but none of my efforts were paying off. I couldn't consistently find reasonable blocks of time in my schedule to go and work out. To make things worse, the long hours sitting at a desk took their toll, and I had pain in my back and legs on a daily basis. Even a new, ergonomic office chair didn't completely solve the pain.

I knew I couldn't keep going on like this, but what could I do? Nothing I tried was working. One day, I came across one of my favorite quotes:

> *"Insanity is doing the same thing over and over and expecting different results."*

I realized I was guilty of the very same thought process and decided to change. I took a step back, analyzed my lifestyle, and listed every excuse I had ever come up with to not exercise. Armed with that list, I was finally prepared to find a solution. Whatever the answer was, it needed to be something that didn't take much time, and preferably could be done throughout the day, instead of all at once. I also wanted to be able to exercise right at, or near, my desk. That meant it would need to be something that didn't require any fancy equipment. Most importantly, it needed to deliver results quickly, before my symptoms got any worse.

Fortunately, I have had a lot of athletic training over the years from the variety of sports and martial arts I studied. I drew upon this experience for ideas and picked training exercises that would potentially fit the specified criteria. After much experimentation and many changes, the first draft of the One Minute Workout System was born.

I was thrilled to find it working better than I had hoped. I was finally working out regularly and before long, the six-pack and other muscles made a welcome reappearance. My core became as strong as steel and the back pain disappeared. In addition, the exercise sessions got me out of the office chair frequently enough that the pain in my legs from sitting too long went away. I felt good again, as though the clock had been turned back ten years. I was able to do all my workouts at home and didn't need to step foot in a gym. And, since I spent so little time working out, I was still able to take care of the other important things in life.

One day I was at the gym visiting my old training buddies and thought, "Why don't I test my strength on the weights?" Despite not training with any free weights or weight machines for over a year, I was quite surprised to find myself stronger than ever. My max bench press went up to 285 pounds, a 40% increase, while my single arm bicep curl went up to 70 pounds, a 75% increase! In addition, I was able to do *one-arm* pull-ups for the first time in my life. Not bad for working out just one or two minutes a day!

A Little About Me

I have been an avid learner for as long as I can remember. Ever since I was a kid, if I found something just a bit interesting, I would do my best to learn as much as I could about it. It didn't matter if it was something simple, like the colorful rocks I found in the backyard, or more complicated, like programming a computer. If something was broken, I always took it apart to see if I could fix it. Nothing was more exciting than the moment where I mastered a new concept or skill. Fortunately, my parents were very supportive, and they fueled my curiosity with ample opportunities to learn new things.

In addition to a variety of intellectual pursuits, I studied music and became a competitive pianist and violinist. The years of training taught me the importance of discipline and consistency when reaching for challenging goals. I also learned a variety of sports such as volleyball, tennis, swimming, gymnastics, figure skating, and martial arts. These experiences gave me a deep understanding of human movement and athletic performance. I hold a black belt in Tae Kwon Do and trained in a variety of styles and weapons in Wushu, or Kung Fu. After success in several martial arts tournaments, I wrote an instructional book on the mechanics of high performance Wushu techniques. Through this book, I was able to share the knowledge and tips that I painstakingly (and painfully!) discovered during my training with other martial artists around the world.

While I was growing up, I found out that I also enjoyed teaching and helping other people. It was extremely satisfying to see other people get that "Aha!" moment when they finally master something they once had trouble with. This, along with my interest in health and fitness, were the reasons I decided to become a doctor instead of an engineer. However, during medical school, I realized that as a doctor, I would only be able to help people one at a time. No matter how many hours I worked, I would only be able to help a tiny portion of the people in the world who needed help. At this point, the engineer in me started looking for ways to find a scalable solution. With my background in computer programming, I started making medical education software to train more healthcare professionals faster.

Helping People Become Healthier

After seeing my results with the One Minute Workout, I wondered how many other people out there are in the same boat as I once was. Even though the details of each person's story are different, the downward spiral that I went through is not unique. What helped me could help many other people. The doctor side of me also started thinking. How many patients had I tried to get started with exercise? How many actually did it? What if this simple system could make more people healthier?

I started thinking about my parents, who are getting older and are far from being in shape. I thought about the countless elderly patients who were admitted to the hospital because of falls. Many of these hospitalizations could have been avoided if they had the strength and balance to protect themselves during the fall, or better yet, to prevent it in the first place. The One Minute Workout is perfect for these people because it is so effective at improving strength, yet simple enough for anybody to follow.

Then I thought, what about people with muscle- and joint-related pains, like my back pain? I have seen so many patients completely dependent on pain killers, from over-the-counter to prescription-only medications, for conditions and injuries with a muscle-related cause. Unfortunately, many of these people rely on medications for symptom relief and never address the underlying cause. There are so many people living with pain that can be lessened through consistent conditioning and increased muscular strength.

Going further, I thought about the ever-increasing number of people who sit down all day at work. How many of us come home and continue to sit in front of a computer, tablet, or television? Research has now shown that sitting for extended periods is so bad for our health, that it is actually killing us. To make it worse, researchers also found that exercising the recommended 30 minutes several times a week fails to prevent, or even reduce, the damage being done. The only way around this silent killer is to get up often. The One Minute Workout gets you out of the chair throughout the day and makes you feel more invigorated from the improved blood flow after doing the short exercises.

Goal: One Million People!

According to the U.S. Center for Disease Control, over one-third of the youth and adults in the United States were overweight or obese in 2011 through 2012, and it continues to get worse. Cases of diabetes and other obesity-related illnesses are also rising. The financial burden on the United States healthcare system from obesity is staggering, estimated at $147 billion in 2008. Unfortunately, this problem is not just limited to the United States. Many countries around the world are also facing the same problem.

So I asked myself … can I get one million people healthier with the One Minute Workout? As these people become stronger and healthier, they would be able to enjoy life better and be happier. This in turn would make the people around them happier as well. Perhaps the prevalence of obesity-related illness and other hospitalizations would go down, decreasing healthcare costs at the same time. Just think of all the tax dollars that could be saved. All this in just one minute day!

With this in mind, I want to share my One Minute Workout System with the world. It has worked so well for me and the people I have told about it. I thought a book would be a great way to tell more people about the One Minute Workout than I could in person. Since I am also an avid computer programmer and technology enthusiast, the One Minute Workout will be available online as a virtual personal trainer service at the OneMinWorkout.com website and in other electronic formats.

However, despite the power of print and technology, nothing compares to hearing it from someone you know and trust. So, if any of your friends or loved ones are at risk from inactivity, obesity, deconditioning, or just plain sitting for too long, please tell them about the One Minute Workout System. Empower them to improve their health. Together, we can reach the goal of one million people!

* * * * * * * *

This book is a work in progress, since I am always learning and trying new things. If you have any comments or suggestions, please feel free to share them with me at *comments@OneMinWorkout.com*. I'd love to learn from you and hear about your experiences.

Introduction

"A workout in just one minute a day?"

"How can one minute be enough to do anything?"

"Is it too good to be true?"

"How does it work?"

"What will it do for me?"

These are probably some of the questions that are going through your head right now. Don't worry, I will answer those questions and a whole lot more. By reading this book, you will learn how to enhance your life with this simple exercise system, which I call the One Minute Workout.

First of all, congratulations on picking up this book. Most of you probably picked it up thinking one of two things—a one minute workout is too good to be true, or a one minute workout is something I need or want. I'm here to tell you that the One Minute Workout (OMW) is an exercise program that truly requires only 60 seconds of your day, and it delivers outstanding results. Whether you hate working out or are already in good shape, the One Minute Workout can lead you to improved fitness, health, appearance, and incredible strength.

Now, you might be a bit skeptical at this point, and for good reason. That's because many of us have been brought up with certain notions about working out. We've been conditioned to think about exercise as something that has to take a lot of time. In fact, it is often seen as a chore. This is because we learn about exercise from people who have been doing it the same way for a long time. When you do something the same way for a long time, you tend to think that is the best way to do it. However, sometimes you need to look at a problem from another perspective to find a better answer. The One Minute Workout will show you a radically different way of working out that takes much less of your valuable time.

We have also been conditioned to think that exercising requires equipment. This is the result of good marketing by fitness equipment companies. New exercise gadgets that promise to tighten your butt or blast your abs come out regularly. Gyms are always advertising their spacious facilities with shiny new exercise machines and weight sets. However, the truth is that none of it is necessary. All you need is your body and some common objects, such as a chair or a couple of books. When used properly, you can get results much faster than you would with all those fancy gadgets. This book will teach you how.

Now, let's talk about what the One Minute Workout is *not*. The One Minute Workout isn't one of those "lose 30 pounds in 7 days" weight loss programs where you gain even more weight afterward. It isn't some new-fangled workout system that you try for a few days and then quit because it's too hard or takes too much time. And for sure, it isn't going to stop global warming or cure cancer.

What the One Minute Workout *will* do is help you make lasting changes to your body and health. It can help you move and feel better, lose fat faster, reduce certain kinds of pain, and improve performance. The One Minute Workout is designed to be an enabler. It enables you to do more with your body than you could before. It can be an end in itself or it can be a stepping stone to bigger and better things, both mental and physical.

The One Minute Workout is for people who want to work out smarter, not just harder. It is a simple exercise system that delivers tremendous results in a small amount of daily exercise time by maximizing every second of your workout. It was carefully engineered to address the most common excuses people give for skipping workouts. This is a system that you can use to improve your health and performance in just one minute a day, no matter what your current level of fitness is. In fact, I would not be surprised if you start feeling better and stronger in as little as one or two weeks.

Do not be fooled by other systems that claim to be "one minute" workouts, but actually require repeating one minute exercise segments many times in a row. Unlike those workouts, the One Minute Workout truly takes only one minute a day.

Here's how it works, in a nutshell:

Each day, you do just *one* exercise from this book. You only need to do that single exercise for a total of one minute for that day. That's it! You don't even need to do the entire minute all at once. You can split it up and do parts of the minute throughout the day. In fact, it's recommended! The next day, you do another exercise for just one minute.

Be assured that this is no joke and there are no gimmicks. The One Minute Workout exercises are designed to fit the constraints of our modern lives. They are specially chosen and organized by difficulty into groups called **Progressions**. When you master one **Exercise** in a Progression, you are ready to move on to the next one. This is how you can keep improving without spending additional time. Even though you will be working out for a short period of time, you will be pushed to your limits. It is a tried and tested exercise system that delivers excellent results.

In just a few chapters, you will learn how to use the One Minute Workout System and why it is so effective. You will also learn how exercise improves your health, fitness, and appearance. Most importantly, you will be able to start exercising right away. By the end of this book, you will have new insight about health and fitness. With this new perspective, I encourage you to come up with your own simple and effective ways to further improve yourself.

How to Use This Book

This book is organized into several sections so that you only need to read the sections that are of interest to you. There is *no need to read it from cover to cover* before beginning your first workout. Below, you'll find a summary of each section in the book so you can easily find the parts that you are interested in.

Quick Start Guide

Flip ahead a few pages to the Quick Start Guide if you want to get started on your first One Minute Workout right away!

Section I: The One Minute Workout

Section I describes the nuts and bolts of the One Minute Workout. You'll learn how a typical day works, what to expect when doing One Minute Workout exercises, and why this exercise system is able to deliver so much in so little workout time. You will also find out how the One Minute Workout can help you target your particular needs.

Section II: Exercise and You

Section II explains how exercise affects your fitness, health, and appearance. You'll learn about the seven components of fitness. Then you will learn about the importance of building muscle, the effect of exercise on specific health conditions, and the dangers of sitting. The last chapter in this section will teach you the factors that affect the appearance of your body and how to use exercise to change them.

Section III: Your Mind and Body

In Section III, you will learn how to set good goals and how to change your habits to achieve those goals. You'll also get tips about eating well, sticking to your plan of action, and maintaining the changes you have made. Chapter 13 goes over muscle anatomy so you understand how your muscles work. Finally, if you have any joint problems or want to improve specific athletic performance, be sure to read "Chapter 14: Fixing Your Body" and "Chapter 15: Improving Your Performance" for workout programming recommendations.

Quick Tip

 For best results, DO NOT leave this book on your bookshelf. If you do so, chances are you'll never open it again and forget about working out. Instead, put it near where you spend most of your time, such as at your desk or by the couch. This way, you will see it often, reminding you to workout.

Sections IV & V: Progressions & Exercises

If you are skipping the earlier sections in the book, be sure to begin with "Chapter 16: Getting Started" so you learn how to do a proper One Minute Workout as well as what to expect when performing these exercises. There are also sample One Minute Workout programs that you can follow. The actual exercises are found in the rest of Section IV and Section V. These sections are designed to be used as a reference so you can quickly find information about each individual exercise.

Remember that in this workout system, related **Exercises** are organized into groups called **Progressions**. The Exercises within each Progression are shown in order of increasing difficulty. This way, you can easily use this book to keep track of your progress through each Progression. Just put a sticky note on the page of the exercise that you are currently working on. When you master an exercise, remove the old sticky note, turn to the next exercise and put a new sticky note on that page for the next time you work on the same Progression.

Section IV contains the **Basic Progressions**, which will help you build a solid foundation of all-around strength. These exercises will not require any special equipment. However, you may use optional equipment to provide variety and additional difficulty.

Section V contains the **Advanced Progressions**, which will dramatically increase your strength and further improve your performance. Most of these advanced exercises will require simple equipment, such as a pull-up bar or a suitable alternative. Be sure to read "Chapter 26: Introduction to the Advanced Progressions" for important details about equipment and tips.

Appendix

In the Appendix, you will find the One Minute Workout Tracker Worksheets and more sample One Minute Workout programs. If you don't want to use the sticky note method, you can use the worksheets to jot down how many seconds of an exercise you do each day. Keeping a record of your workout efforts will keep you organized and, just as importantly, keep you motivated. All you have to do is look over your workout records to see how far you have come. There is no greater motivation than knowing that you are on the right track and that your efforts are paying off.

3

Quick Start Guide

All right, so you're eager to get started with your first One Minute Workout. Let's begin with an exercise from the Basic Progressions to give you a taste of what the One Minute Workout is about.

Using a stable chair, try holding one of the exercise positions shown below for as long as you can. Count or use a clock to time yourself. Stop when you get tired or when 60 seconds is up, whichever comes first. You should feel the muscles in your arms, chest, upper back, abs, and hip flexors strongly engaged during this exercise.

Rising Chair Press
(Feet On Ground)

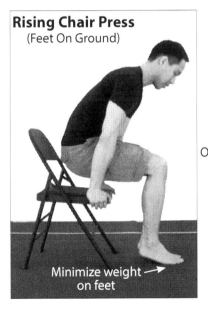

Minimize weight → on feet

OR

Tuck Sit Press
(Feet Off Ground)

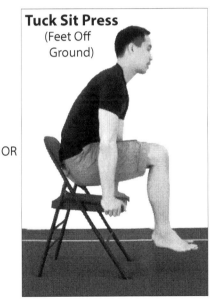

Rising Chair Press: *While sitting, place your hands by your thighs. Raise your butt off the chair by pressing down on the chair with your hands while keeping your elbows straight. Your feet can touch the floor lightly to provide some support but don't push down on the floor. Keep most of your body weight on your hands.*

Tuck Sit Press: *The same as the Rising Chair Press, but lift your feet off the ground by squeezing your abs and hip flexors.*

Write down the number of seconds you held the exercise here _____.

Didn't make it to the end of the full minute? That's all right! That means the exercise was appropriately difficult for you. The beauty of the One Minute Workout is that you can finish the rest of the 60 seconds throughout the day. If you were able to complete the entire minute just now, then you're ready to take on a more difficult exercise from the Sit Press Progression found in Section IV.

Whether you finished a whole minute or not, chances are your abs started burning or your arms started shaking while doing the above exercise. That's proof that your muscles were getting an intense work-out. In just those few seconds, you blasted your chest, shoulders, arms, back, abs, and hip flexors all at the same time. That's almost your whole body! This is why the One Minute Workout can deliver so much in so little time.

By doing one of these appropriately difficult exercises for one minute each day, I am certain you'll notice a difference in as little as one to two weeks. You'll feel stronger than on day one, be able to hold the exercise position longer, and maybe even notice that you can move and do things better. People have excitedly told me how just this one exercise helped them move and feel better, improve their golf swing, or reduce their chronic back pain, among other things. Imagine how much more benefit you can gain from doing the other exercises in this book.

As you keep doing an exercise from the One Minute Workout, you'll get stronger and be able to master it by doing the exercise for a full continuous minute. At that point, you're ready to move on to the next Exercise in the Progression. Now, you're using the One Minute Workout *System*.

What makes the One Minute Workout System truly effective is how easy it is to stick with. Exercise only does your body good when you do it consistently. But, that's the hardest part for most people. I had the same problem. That's why making the workout system as easy to stick with as possible was my most important goal. Just one exercise, one minute a day. No gyms, no special equipment, no sweating required.

You can get an effective workout anytime you have just a few seconds, practically anywhere you may be. With such convenience, you now have ZERO excuses not to get in shape!

Now that you've had a taste of your first One Minute Workout, it's time to learn more about the system and what to expect from here. Go to Section I to learn more about the One Minute Workout System. For more information on exercise and health and for diet tips, read Sections II and III. Or, feel free to jump straight to Section IV for the One Minute Workout exercises and workout plans.

All right! If you haven't finished your whole minute of the Sit Press exercise, now is a great time to put in a few more seconds. Then, take a break, explore more of this book, or go do something fun. Just remember to do more exercise sessions later on, until you reach a total of 60 seconds for the day. At that point, you'll have completed your first full minute of the day in the One Minute Workout System.

Section I

The
One Minute Workout

4

How It Works

The One Minute Workout System is unlike any other workout system out there. All you need is just one minute a day and you'll be on your way to better fitness and health. Designed with busy people in mind, the One Minute Workout delivers big gains in the least amount of workout time.

The core of the One Minute Workout revolves around the specially selected exercises in the system. These exercises use your body weight for resistance, so you can perform them virtually anytime and anywhere. **Exercises** that are related to each other are organized into groups called **Progressions**. Each progression focuses on a different set of muscles in a particular movement, so even though the muscle groups targeted in one progression may overlap with those targeted by another progression, the muscles are worked differently in each one. This intentional overlap is one of the reasons that you can make massive progress with just one exercise per day. For example, the Sit Press

---

One Minute Workout Terms

Exercise: The activity that you do to train your body.

Progression: A group of related Exercises that are ordered by difficulty.

Exercise Session: The actual performance of an Exercise. For example, holding a Tuck Sit Press would be one Session.

Master an Exercise: Complete the entire minute of the Exercise all in a single session.

Supercharge an Exercise: To do more than a total of one minute of the Exercise in one day.

Progression focuses mostly on your upper body while the Squat Progression focuses on the legs. However, they both work on the muscles in your core.

The exercises in each progression are ordered by increasing difficulty. Which exercise you should use from each progression depends on your current strength level. For example, if you are just starting out, you might start with the first exercise in a progression. These are generally easy enough that anybody can do them. On the other hand, if you are in better shape, you might start with an exercise somewhere in the middle of the progression. As you get stronger and master the exercise, you are ready to move up to the next exercise in the progression. This increases the difficulty so that you can continue to train your body just as intensely as before in the same amount of workout time. The most difficult exercises in each progression are challenging even for those who are very strong and in excellent shape.

The Workout Routine

Each day, you pick a different progression to focus on and perform just the one exercise from that progression appropriate for your strength level. By picking a different progression for each day, you target your muscles differently. The goal is to do that exercise for a total of one minute for that day. Just 60 seconds, and you're done for the day!

You don't need to complete the minute all at once. You can split it up throughout the day into several **exercise sessions**. In fact, this is the way you will end up doing the exercises on most days, because an exercise of the appropriate difficulty is one that you are not yet able to do continuously for a full minute. Each time you do an exercise, that is considered an exercise session, regardless of how many seconds it is. For example, doing a Front Plank for 10 seconds in a row is one session, as is doing it for 20 or 30 seconds in a row.

For each exercise session, do the exercise for as long as you can. Don't be afraid to push yourself, since doing so is how you improve. If you haven't accumulated a total of sixty seconds of that exercise for the day, just do more sessions throughout the day until you do. Over time, you will get stronger and be able to do the exercise for longer periods of time, decreasing the number of sessions it takes to finish the minute for the day.

Keep in mind that as you work on each exercise, your goal is to extend the length of your exercise sessions so that you eventually **master** the exercise. Mastering an exercise means that you can perform it for an entire minute in a single session. This indicates that you are strong enough to advance to a more difficult exercise in the progression. The next day that you come back to the same progression, you can start working on the next exercise. There is no need to keep working on the exercises you have already mastered.

If you are feeling adventurous or want to progress faster, you can try **supercharging** your exercises. That means doing a particular exercise for more than a total of one minute for the day. Supercharging is completely optional and not necessary for the regular One Minute Workout System.

A typical workout in a day might look something like this:

1. Pick the progression you want to do for the day. The exercise that you are working on in this progression is your exercise for the day (e.g. Tuck Sit Press from the Sit Press Progression).
2. Do a 20-second exercise session in the morning before breakfast.
3. Go to work.
4. While sitting at your computer at work, do another 20-second exercise session.
5. Leave work and go home.
6. Do the last 20-second exercise session during a commercial break while watching TV. That's a total of 60 seconds. You're done for the day!

As you see, you can do your exercise sessions almost any time you want. You can spread them throughout the day as in the example above, or you can group them in one part of the day. Do them whenever you have a little down time or when you need a break. It is totally up to you. Just make sure you finish a total of one minute before the end of the day. Here are some ideas for when you can do an exercise:

1. After you wake up.
2. During a coffee or snack break.
3. Before a meal.
4. While waiting in line.
5. While watching TV.
6. During a commercial break.
7. At work during a short break.
8. Surfing the Web or watching online videos (great during pre-roll ads).
9. Waiting for the train or bus.
10. At the gym (if you are already there).

Whatever your schedule, the general flow for each day will look something like the flowchart below.

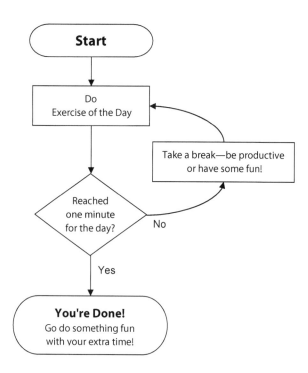

With the One Minute Workout, you won't need to drive to the gym, you won't need to change into workout clothes, and you won't need to shower afterward. How's that for saving even more time?

You may have come across other workout systems that claim to be "one minute" workouts. Don't be tricked! They usually ask you to do multiple sets of one minute exercise intervals in a row, often mixed with many more minutes of lower intensity "recovery" exercises. These workouts end up being much longer than one minute and usually run ten, twenty or even thirty minutes. They are certainly not one minute workouts.

What Equipment Will I Need?

The One Minute Workout system requires almost no specialized equipment. You won't need a set of weights, workout machines, or fancy gadgets. In general, all you will need is some floor space and perhaps a chair, some books, or other similar objects. The only time you may need specialized equipment is if you want to do the Advanced Progressions, some of which require a support to hang from, such as a pull-up bar or ledge, and perhaps exercise rings or suspension trainers. You may choose to use some aids to ease hand positions, or to add resistance, but the One Minute Workout is designed with simplicity in mind. You can find more details about optional and suggested equipment in "Chapter 16: Getting Started" and "Chapter 26: Introduction to the Advanced Progressions" from Section IV and Section V respectively.

How Static Exercises Work

The exercises in the One Minute Workout are all *static exercises*. This means that once you get into position, you don't move until you are done with the exercise session. The act of holding the position is the exercise itself. For example, in a Tuck Sit Press, you lift your body off the chair using only your hands, and hold that position until you are done. This is in contrast to dynamic exercises such as push-ups and sit-ups in which you are always moving.

Now, you might be wondering how your muscles are getting a work-out if they don't move. Holding your body in these exercise positions requires your muscles to be engaged and puts them under a load. This load is what gives your muscles a workout and stimulates them to grow stronger in response. In fact, you may be surprised how much of a workout it can be. For example, just try squatting halfway down to the ground and holding that position. I bet you will feel the burn in your leg muscles before long.

Since static exercises do not involve repeated movement, we need to measure them differently. Instead of counting repetitions like you would in a dynamic exercise, you count how long the static position is held. Holding static exercise for longer times is like doing more repetitions of a dynamic exercise. They both mean that the target muscles have been worked out more. This is why the One Minute Workout is all about doing the exercises for a set amount of time, rather than repetitions.

How the Progressions Work

Your body is amazingly efficient at adapting to stresses placed on it. For example, when weight training, you need to keep increasing the weight and the number of repetitions because your body adapts by becoming stronger and more efficient. By continuously challenging your body, you can make incredible improvements. However, the instant you stop challenging your body, progress slows down and stops.

People often ask me, "How do the exercises in each progression get harder without the use of weights or other similar equipment?" Good question! The One Minute Workout takes advantage of biomechanics and uses something I call *reverse leverage*, which is mechanical leverage *against* your muscles. Even though your body weight doesn't change, you can increase the load placed on your muscles during an exercise by changing your body position in specific ways. This increases the training resistance and makes you stronger, similar to using heavier weights. As you get stronger and move on to more difficult exercises in a progression, your body position is changed again to increase the training resistance. This is why related exercises are organized into progressions.

By adjusting the amount of leverage, the effective load on the target muscles can range from as little as a fraction of your body weight to several times it. This means you are essentially a walking gym!

In the chapters detailing each progression, you will find my recommendations for which exercise to start with based on your current fitness level. If you find a continuous minute of the suggested exercise too easy, try a harder one. Similarly, if you find it too hard to even get started, try an easier one. An appropriate exercise is one that you can do for at least five seconds, but less than one minute. Five seconds is generally the minimum amount of time for an exercise to be effective.

If you are on the easiest exercise in a progression but still can't hold it for five seconds, then hold it for as long as you can, even if it is only one second. Keep doing as many of these short holds as you can each time you work out. This will help increase your strength. Soon, you will be able to hold the position for longer periods of time, and eventually you will build up enough strength to hold it for five seconds.

* * * * * * * *

This covers the basics of how the One Minute Workout System works. Keep in mind that the One Minute Workout is a system, not just a workout. Once you get started, follow the system until you get the results you desire. It really doesn't get any easier than this. Just one minute a day, anytime, anywhere, and no sweating needed. Now there's no excuse not to be in shape!

The next chapter explains the principles of why the One Minute Workout System works. If you want to start working out right away, you can skip ahead to "Chapter 16: Getting Started" in Section IV.

⏱ 5
Why It Works

The One Minute Workout System is the most time-efficient and effective workout system you will ever try. Despite such short workout times, it can deliver big results because it leverages biomechanics and logistics through the following four principles:

1. **MITI Principle (pronounced like "mighty")**
2. **Massive Muscle Engagement**
3. **Convenience**
4. **Sustainability**

These principles ensure that you get the most physiological benefit in the smallest amount of workout time. Furthermore, they make this a workout that takes much less willpower and effort to do and maintain. This means the One Minute Workout is an easy way for you to effectively improve your life regardless of what your current fitness level and schedule may be.

1. The MITI Principle

The One Minute Workout system uses specific bodyweight exercises that are static. These specially selected exercises utilize the **Maximum Intensity Training Interval (MITI)** principle. As the name suggests, it means working the target muscles at maximum intensity for the entire training interval. For example, if you close your hand and squeeze as tightly as you can, your hand muscles are working as hard as they can the entire time. Similarly, when you do a MITI exercise, your muscles are loaded to full capacity for the entire duration of the exercise. Therefore MITI exercises are very time-efficient ways to work your muscles and build strength.

Dynamic exercises, which are usually repetitive, do not utilize the MITI principle because the movement itself changes the load on your muscles. For example, a push-up movement loads your chest muscles and triceps differently depending on the angle of your elbows and shoulders. At the top of a push-up, they face the least amount of load. In fact, this is almost a resting position. When you lower your body down near the floor, the triceps and pectorals face the highest load. When you push your body back up, the load on your muscles decrease again. So over the duration of the exercise, your muscles are worked much less compared to a MITI exercise. Figure 1 shows the exercise intensity for one repetition of a push-up. Note how the intensity varies as you go through the movement.

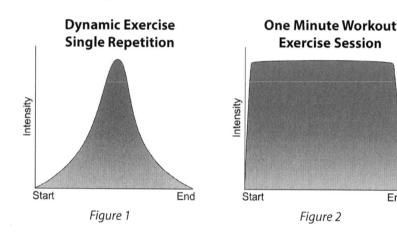

Figure 1

Figure 2

On the other hand, static exercises do not move once you get in position. Therefore, your muscles experience the same load for the duration of the exercise. Take a look at Figure 2 representing a MITI exercise session from the One Minute Workout. The shaded area represents how much intensity your muscles experience throughout the exercise. Note how much larger the shaded area is in this graph compared to the one on the left.

Furthermore, when performing a static exercise, there is no movement and therefore no momentum. You can't "cheat" and use momentum to help you complete a movement like you could in a dynamic exercise. If you've ever lifted weights before, you probably noticed how much easier it is to lift it by swinging it into position. The slower you lift it, the harder it is. While using momentum makes it easier to complete a repetition, this "cheat" is undesirable, since it reduces the intensity your muscles experience, and therefore the effectiveness of the exercise. In a way, you can think of a static exercise as being so slow that it doesn't move. Without the aid of momentum, you ensure that your muscles get the most out of the exercise.

You might ask, "What if I do several repetitions of a dynamic exercise?" While your muscles will definitely get more of a workout, it still doesn't compare with a MITI exercise performed for the same amount of time. Dynamic repetitions are generally short, on the order of a few seconds at most (Figure 3). The sum of the time your muscles spend fully engaged during each repetition is still less than the time they spend engaged during a One Minute Workout MITI exercise (Figure 4). One Minute Workout exercises essentially compress all of the intensity your muscles would experience from traditional dynamic exercises into just one minute. This is a major reason why the One Minute Workout System is so time-efficient and effective.

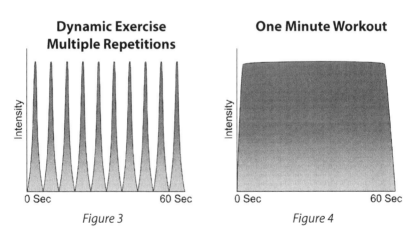

Figure 3   Figure 4

It is important to keep in mind that not every static exercise is a MITI exercise. It depends on whether that particular exercise is appropriate for your strength level at that time. You have to make sure that the exercise works your target muscles to 100% of their capacity. If you are doing an exercise that is too easy, then it is not a MITI exercise for you. So, a particular exercise may be MITI for somebody else but not necessarily for you. Similarly, an exercise that was MITI for you at one point will no longer be as you get stronger.

In the One Minute Workout, the exercises in each progression get harder and harder. By advancing through these progressions as you get stronger, you will always be doing an exercise that loads your muscles to their full capacity. This way, you can continue to reap the benefits of MITI training, no matter how strong you get.

While there are many benefits to static exercises, one of the weaknesses of static exercises is that the majority of strength improvement is limited to a small range of movement around the position that was trained. The One Minute Workout System overcomes this problem by using the concept of progressions. As you work through a progression, you work through a large part of your entire movement range. Different progressions also work your muscles in different directions. In this way, the One Minute Workout System greatly increases your strength throughout your range of motion.

2. Massive Muscle Engagement

Many traditional exercises target individual muscles, or just a few muscles at the same time. For example, bicep curls focus mostly on the biceps, while sit-ups focus on the abs and possibly some of the hip flexors. With these traditional exercises, you have to do many different exercises to train all of the different muscles.

In contrast, *compound exercises* involve multiple joints and muscle groups. This means you can work on many more muscles in the same amount of time. All of the One Minute Workout (OMW) exercises engage multiple joints and muscle groups simultaneously. Some exercises involve nearly the entire body! Therefore, you can do just one OMW exercise a day and still train a large number of muscle groups.

Another way that the One Minute Workout achieves massive muscle engagement is by employing exercises that incorporate the element of balance. When you perform exercises that require balance, you work on all of the muscles that help you maintain your balance. This means you train antagonistic muscle pairs simultaneously, such as the biceps and triceps, since one muscle compensates for overcorrections by its opposing muscle.

Also, many of the OMW exercises use *reverse leverage*. This means many more of your muscles need to be engaged in order to support and to stabilize your joints during these exercises. Much like the guy-wires on a radio tower or utility pole, your muscles maintain tension in different directions on a joint and keep it from moving too far in any one direction. All of the muscles acting on a joint will be engaged regardless of the direction of the main training load. This means that you build strength even faster. Just as importantly, you will also develop the ability to protect your joints from injury.

One Minute Workout exercises focus largely on strengthening the core muscles, which include the abdominal, lower back, and oblique muscles. All of the exercises in this system work on the core, thereby ensuring that it becomes strong enough to handle your specific body mechanics. This means you don't have to spend extra time on core-specific exercises. It is automatically taken care of with your daily OMW exercise.

3. Convenience

Getting ready to go work out is half the battle. How often have you thought about the gym but end up not going? You probably told yourself that you'll skip the workout just this one time. The only problem is that one time becomes two, then two becomes three. Before you know it, you no longer work out.

The One Minute Workout solves this problem through convenience. Since many of the exercises in this system do not require any special equipment, you can do them virtually anytime and anywhere. This saves you a lot of time going to and from the gym, changing clothes, waiting for your turn, setting up the equipment, etc. You can literally do your One Minute Workout exercise at your desk, on the couch, or even in the elevator. They are so simple to do that there really aren't any excuses for not doing them.

Earlier, you learned how the One Minute Workout leverages biomechanics to deliver so much in so little workout time. Combined with the convenience of doing these exercises anytime and anywhere, the

One Minute Workout saves you even more time. In the same 30 minutes spent at a gym, you could have done a whole month's worth of working out with the One Minute Workout!

However, it gets even better. Since you can break up the One Minute Workout throughout the day, it is even easier to squeeze in an exercise session here and there. In a traditional workout, you usually do sets of repetitions with rest breaks between sets. If you are at the gym, you can't really do much else while resting. However, if you are at your desk, or by the TV, you can do your exercise and get right back to what you were doing earlier, whether it was being productive or having a good time. The "resting" time can be spent doing something useful instead of waiting around at the gym. This is another great benefit of the One Minute Workout which further enables you to maximize the use of your time.

Even if you get so busy that you forget to finish the minute for the day, doing part of the minute is still much better than nothing at all. This happened to me at first. That's why I made some online tools to make it even easier to stay on track. We'll talk about these tools a bit later in the chapter.

4. Sustainability

Often, the hardest part of exercising is getting started. This is where many people get stuck. The idea of being in shape and looking great is enticing, but taking the first step can be daunting. Some workout programs require specialized training before you can get started safely (e.g. Olympic weightlifting). Others, such as boot camps, push you so hard in the beginning that you don't feel like doing it ever again. However, the exercises in the One Minute Workout system start out so easy that virtually anyone can do them. As you get stronger, you progress at your own pace to harder exercises. If you are already in great shape, you can always start with the harder exercises and progress from there.

Once you start exercising, the next most difficult part is making sure you do it regularly. Regardless of which workout system you use, if you don't do it, it won't work. When people stop working out, they usually give common excuses, such as lack of time or difficulty accessing equipment. All of these reasons contribute to something I call *workout fatigue*. I'm not talking about getting physically tired, but rather, losing motivation. The higher the barriers are to working out, the more willpower and effort it takes to go work out. This means you will be less likely to keep doing it over time. The One Minute Workout breaks down many of these barriers, so it takes less willpower and discipline to get started and stay on track.

Workout fatigue also sets in when you work out but don't notice any progress. Who wants to keep doing something when they don't seem to get anything out of it? This isn't a problem with the One Minute Workout because progress is constantly measured and easy to see. Since you measure your exercise duration every session, you will always know where you stand. If you can do an exercise for longer than before, then you are making progress even if it is only one second more. If you master an exercise, then you are making progress.

With traditional exercises, doing one more repetition than your current record often requires a sizable improvement in strength and endurance. Until you improve enough, you will be stuck at the same number of repetitions. Without seeing an increase in the repetition count, it is easy to feel like you aren't making any progress. This rarely happens with the One Minute Workout because progress is measured in much smaller increments. It is easier to focus and perform an exercise for just a little longer than before, compared to doing another repetition of a dynamic exercise. While these improvements may seem small at first, it is measurable and real progress. Those additional seconds will add up quickly, and before you know it, you will have mastered that exercise.

Making *measurable progress* is the key to beating workout fatigue. It is the one thing that can keep you motivated despite the barriers. If you see that you are making enough progress for the amount of effort you put in, then you will be more likely to stick with it. Unfortunately, this is a weakness of many other workout systems. Some just don't deliver any visible results to keep you going. Others fail to measure it in a way that makes it easily noticeable. Without measurable progress, chances are that you will quit before long.

If for some reason you get off track and find yourself forgetting to do your OMW exercises, it's easy to restart. Even if you stop working out for so long that you get out of shape again, getting back into the One Minute Workout is as simple as getting started in the first place.

* * * * * * * *

The One Minute Workout is highly effective because of the biomechanics and convenience of its exercises. This lowers the barriers to exercise as much as possible, making it a sustainable workout system that anyone can start and maintain. By doing the One Minute Workout regularly, you can make dramatic improvements in your fitness, health, appearance, and performance.

Using a Reminder System

When I first started using the One Minute Workout, it worked really well. But on some days, I was so busy trying to get as much done as possible, I would forget to do the exercises throughout the day, even for a few seconds. As a result, I would cram the entire minute in before bed. However, I still wasn't getting out of the office chair as much as I had originally hoped. To solve this, I created a simple reminder system to keep myself on track. Each time a reminder popped up on my cell phone, I would stop what I was doing and do an exercise session. If I couldn't take a break at that instant, I was still much more likely to remember to do it after completing the task at hand. After seeing how well the reminders worked, I developed the reminder system further to integrate it with the One Minute Workout System. The result is the virtual personal trainer software mentioned earlier, which I now use every day.

If you find yourself getting off track, you can use a reminder system to motivate yourself. Just pick one that you find easy to use, or use the virtual personal trainer service on the One Minute Workout website, which features a custom-built reminder system that takes the thinking out of working out. Go to www.OneMinWorkout.com for more information.

What About Cardio?

When people talk about cardio exercises, they are commonly referring to aerobic, or endurance, exercises. Due to the physiology of our bodies, aerobic exercises require time. You need to work your muscles long enough to get past the anaerobic phase and into the aerobic phase. The anaerobic phase can last anywhere from a few seconds up to a minute or so, depending on the particular muscle and level of conditioning. One Minute Workouts are not aerobic exercises. You won't feel tired or winded in the same way as you would running, but they will get your heart rate up. In fact, you just might be surprised to find yourself slightly out of breath after an exercise session.

Traditional cardio exercises use long periods of low to moderate intensity exercises to get your heart rate up. In contrast, the One Minute Workout exercises get your heart rate up using high intensity activity over short periods of time. When OMW exercise sessions are done in a short amount of time, they become a form of high intensity interval training, which confers cardiovascular benefits as well. They won't replace traditional cardio training, but if you're short on time, you will get a wider range of benefits from the One Minute Workout exercises. In addition, by using the exercise sessions to break up your sitting time throughout the day, you will help protect your health from the dangerous effects of prolonged sitting. This is something cardio workouts won't protect you from, even if you do them the recommended three times per week or more.

○⏱ 6
Who Is This For?

First, let's talk about who the One Minute Workout is NOT for. It is not for people who like to spend hours at the gym. It is not for people who enjoy slaving away at the treadmill. And, it is not for people who have no desire to improve their health and lives. If you sound like any of these people, you can put this book down and keep doing whatever you have been doing. Don't worry, you'll continue to get the same results you've already been getting.

So, who is the One Minute Workout for? The OMW is for people who don't have a lot of time. It is for people who think going to the gym is a hassle. It is for people who want to increase their strength so that they can be more active and reduce the chance of injuries. It is for people who want to enhance their athletic performance by accelerating their rate of improvement. It is for people who want to improve their bodies so that they can lead healthier and more productive lives. The One Minute Workout is a system to help people get in better functional shape so they can focus on getting the most out of life without spending more of it in the gym.

I designed the One Minute Workout to enhance many aspects of fitness simultaneously. It is great as a stand-alone workout system, or in combination with another workout routine to accelerate your progress. Since the One Minute Workout only takes one minute a day, it is extremely easy to add to your daily schedule or workout routine. Go through the flowchart on the next two pages to see how the One Minute Workout can help you. Or take a look at the common situations listed afterward to find out what the OMW System can do for you.

Is the One Minute Workout Right For You?

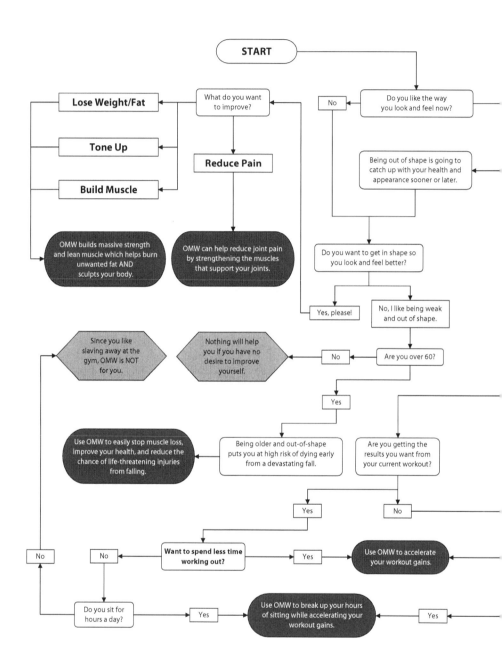

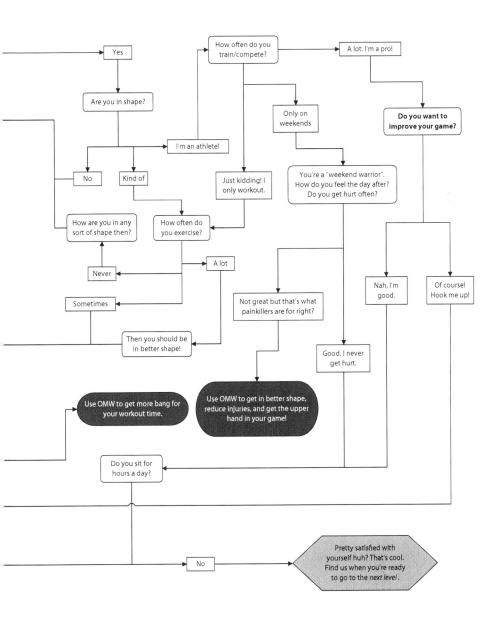

I am a(n):

Couch Potato

Right now, you're not very active. You want to be, but it's hard to get yourself started on any sort of workout program. This could be because you lack enough energy, time, or other resources. Also, any sort of physical activity feels like hard work. Your muscles are weak, your joints are weak, and you're probably gaining weight. Unfortunately, this sedentary lifestyle is silently killing you.

The One Minute Workout System can help you turn this all around. Your weakness is low motivation. However, this simple and convenient workout system takes so little time that you have no excuses not to do it. You are going to gain strength, and your functional movement will improve, making any physical activity easier. It is also a great way to break up long periods of sitting so that you can be healthier. Who knows, once you start doing these exercises, you might even want to be more active!

Desk Worker

You have a job where you are sitting most of the day. In fact, you might even have back or leg pain from sitting so much. And, if you didn't already know, those hours of sitting at the desk are literally killing you. You try your best to work out before or after work, but you don't seem to be getting the results you want. Or, you wish you could spend less time working out but still get results.

The One Minute Workout System can help get you out of the chair throughout the day and make your body stronger at the same time. You are going to feel better and be more productive after these micro-breaks. Your bodily pains may also improve as your core gets stronger. You might even find yourself looking forward to taking more of these healthy breaks. If that's the case, go right ahead—you don't have to stop at just one minute! With these short workouts throughout the day, you won't need to spend so much time at the gym anymore.

Weekend Warrior

Weekend warriors are what we call people who can't or don't work out regularly during the week but jump into vigorous activities on the weekends. You aren't really in shape, but you play hard anyway. Unfortunately, it is not uncommon for you to start the new work week feeling sore all over, and possibly sporting a brace or wrap for an injury you got over the weekend.

The One Minute Workout will free you from this cycle of inactivity and overactivity. It will toughen up your entire body so that you'll be able to go several games with your buddies and still feel like a champ the day after. It'll also bring your game up a few notches by increasing your strength and improving your fundamental fitness level.

Athlete

You are an active competitor and you train to win. As an athlete, you are looking to improve your performance as fast as possible. While each sport requires a unique set of skills, all sports require strong fundamentals. This means coordinating a well-rounded foundation of strength to generate power, and then transferring it efficiently throughout your body.

The One Minute Workout builds tremendous strength, body awareness, and balance that will accelerate the gains you get from your regular training. Since it only takes an extra minute a day, it's a no-brainer for any serious athlete!

Older Person (> 60 Years Old)

As an older person, your priorities are different. In the latter third of life, wear and tear catches up to you. Your body no longer works as well as it used to. However, you desire to retain your ability to be active, despite the ongoing muscle loss that comes with age. You also want to be able to protect yourself from the dreaded falls and life-threatening injuries that can accompany them.

The One Minute Workout is a simple way to build strength and prevent muscle loss, all in the comfort of your home. It will also enhance your sense of balance, so that you'll be less likely to fall. And in the event that you do take a tumble, you'll be better prepared to protect yourself from injury.

* * * * * * * *

If you aren't one of those people, then you might be looking to do some of the following:

I Want to Tone My Muscles

One Minute Workouts build dense, lean muscles, right where you want them. This system will help you get a core of steel and define all of your muscles. Tighten up that butt, trim up those arms, and build six-pack abs!

I Want to Lose Weight

It's important to be healthy for your weight. However, you want to make sure you lose fat weight, not just water or muscle weight. You may not lose fifty pounds right away with the One Minute Workout, but it will help you become a healthier version of you, whatever weight you're naturally meant to be.

I Want to Lose Flab

The One Minute Workout system is an ultra-easy way to build lean muscle that will accelerate all of your fat loss efforts. And when the fat is gone, the sexy muscles will already be there for everyone to see!

I Want to Maintain My Physique

You worked hard to get the body you already have, but you don't need to keep slaving away at the gym to maintain it. Use this simple system to keep all of your hard-earned muscles, all in just one minute a day.

I Want to Build Massive Muscles

To build big bulky muscles, you need to lift big, heavy weights. The One Minute Workout System isn't designed to make you look like the Hulk, but it will still make you massively stronger, so that you can lift even bigger, heavier weights. Use OMW in addition to your current training regimen and you'll be able to bulk up faster than ever before.

* * * * * * * *

Did you find something in this chapter that sounds like you? If so, now you know why you need the One Minute Workout. If not, don't worry. In the next chapter, we'll go into more detail about what the One Minute Workout can do for you. After learning about the benefits of OMW, you can decide if it is right for you.

What It Does for You

Now that you know how and why the One Minute Workout works and who it is designed for, it's time to find out exactly what it does for you. Even though the One Minute Workout is a simple workout system, it imparts several important benefits. These benefits improve your ability to move and function. As a result of these changes, your health and appearance will improve as well.

Some of the specific benefits you can get from using the One Minute Workout are:

- Increased Functional Strength
- Enhanced Balance
- Fat and/or Weight Loss
- Increased Lean Muscle
- Improved Muscle Tone and Appearance
- Reduced Musculoskeletal-Related Pain

Increasing Functional Strength

At the fundamental level, strength is the basis of all movement. Without sufficient strength, you cannot do even the simplest things, like getting up to go to the bathroom, grooming and dressing yourself, preparing your meals, or other similar *activities of daily living*. This is why you need to continually maintain, and ideally improve, your strength. As it increases, the things you can already do become easier, and the range of activities you are capable of broadens. This means you can try things you weren't able to do before. It is for this reason, the One Minute Workout System focuses on building strength, especially functional strength.

What exactly is functional strength? *Functional strength* is useful strength. You want strength that helps your body perform the practical movements in your daily life, such as those related to your job, household, or even the sports you play.

For example, when lifting your child or a heavy box of tools, you squat down then stand up. To do this, you need squatting strength, not just quad or hamstring strength. Similarly, when you push things around, such as a heavy shopping cart or a lawn mower, you need plank strength to keep your core rigid so you can effectively transfer force from your legs to your arms. This kind of functional strength also helps with your overall posture, whether you are standing or sitting. Another example is when you climb or pull things around. Here, you need pulling strength. All of these functional movements utilize multiple muscle groups throughout the body. So, when you build functional strength, you work on multiple muscle groups at the same time. In addition, you also learn to better coordinate them to produce useful movement.

On the other hand, exercises that isolate a single muscle group generally do not develop much functional strength. The bicep curl is a great example. This is a classic exercise that people do at the gym because big biceps give the impression of great strength. However, very few useful movements solely use the biceps. When you pick up a bag of groceries or a heavy box, you're not just engaging your biceps. You also need to use your upper back and shoulder muscles, as well as your core. I'm not saying exercises like this aren't good for you. Since these exercises focus on each muscle separately, you'll just need to spend more time and effort to do more exercises in order to get the same functional benefits.

The One Minute Workout delivers great functional benefit in a short time through bodyweight exercises that train multiple muscle groups simultaneously. Working with your body weight and shape teaches you how to manage your body effectively. This is one of the key principles behind the OMW exercises. Training with OMW increases your functional strength, enabling you to be more active while reducing your chances of getting hurt.

Improving Your Balance

If you have difficulty with activities in your daily life, functional strength is only one part of the problem. The other part is balance, which is a combination of body awareness and compensatory strength. Skilled athletes have honed their body awareness and conditioned their muscles so that they have a keen sense of balance. They are able to respond quickly and appropriately in order to prevent injury. For the amount of physical activity they do, their rate of injury is actually quite low.

On the other end of the spectrum, people who are deconditioned, or out-of-shape, are at higher risk of falling and getting injured. These people usually have decreased body awareness and lack the compensatory strength necessary to adjust their balance quickly. When they fall, they don't have enough strength to protect themselves from the impact. As a result, they sustain more serious injuries than they would have if they were in better physical shape.

Who tends to be deconditioned? Older people, especially those over the age of 60, are often deconditioned, since they have been losing muscle mass for many years. People who have been sick for a while are also usually deconditioned. You may be surprised to hear that it only takes a day or two of bed rest to start losing muscle mass. This also happens if you are inactive for several days, but to a lesser degree. Therefore, people who have sedentary jobs and don't exercise much are often deconditioned. Fortunately, much of this muscle loss can be prevented by simply getting up and doing some light exercise.

The One Minute Workout System uses bodyweight exercises that help train your sense of balance and improve body awareness. As you work on these aspects, you will learn how to use your body better and gain the strength necessary to correct your balance quickly and appropriately.

Losing Fat and/or Weight

Many people want to lose weight and fat to improve their health and body image. While the two may seem like the same thing, losing weight and losing fat are two very different goals. One is about being healthy for your body type, and the other is mostly mental. As we will cover in "Chapter 9: Improving Your Health Through Exercise," you should be more concerned with losing fat, since that is what affects your health and the way you look. Don't be overly concerned with your weight, especially when you gain muscle. Muscle weighs more than fat, and as you get more of it, you may still weigh the same or even a little more, even as the fat gradually disappears. This is normal and to be expected.

The One Minute Workout is designed to build strength and lean muscle mass. As you will learn later on, lean muscle helps you burn fat faster. It burns more calories at rest and even more when you move around. More muscle mass also makes movement easier, making you more likely to be active and burn additional calories.

Building Lean Muscle and Improving Muscle Tone and Appearance

Since the One Minute Workout exercises build strong, lean muscles, your muscles will become more defined. This will improve the way you look because your muscles will have increased volume and more contours to shape your body. Building muscle also helps you lose fat faster, which will allow those contours to show through even better.

Reducing Musculoskeletal-Related Pain

Ever throw out your back? You were probably laid up for a week or longer. Many musculoskeletal pains come about from injuries caused by weak muscles. The culprits are often the core and other supporting muscles that are frequently ignored. It doesn't matter how big your chest, biceps, or legs are if your core is weak. Your body moves by transferring power from one part of the body to another part through the core. Without a strong core, you are unable to transfer power safely and efficiently, thereby increasing your chances of getting hurt. Therefore, it stands to reason that the strongest part of your body should be your core.

The same goes for other joints, such as the knees, shoulders, elbows, etc. Without strong supporting muscles, your joints face excessive levels of stress, which wear them out faster and can cause injury. Strengthening the supporting muscles is an effective way to reduce these stresses, improve joint function, and reduce joint pain. In fact, this is the basis of many physical rehabilitation programs.

One Minute Workout exercises focus intensely on developing core strength, so that your core will become an asset, not a weakness. As those muscles gain strength and become balanced, you may find a reduction in pain-related issues in your back and other muscles. You may also find that OMW exercises help with other common trouble muscle groups and joints, such as the rotator cuff and knees. I know they did for me. After using the One Minute Workout for a while, my back pain essentially vanished and my shoulders felt a lot better and more stable.

Section II

Exercise and You

⏱ 8
What Is Fitness?

Our bodies can do amazing things, but only when taken care of. Unfortunately, the pressures of modern life leave many of us with little time or energy to give our bodies the care they deserve. The result is that many people have physical pain and largely preventable health problems, such as obesity, cardiovascular disease, and diabetes. These medical conditions put a tremendous burden on us personally, as well as our healthcare system. Wouldn't it be great if there was something that could help solve all of these problems?

The good news is that there is. It's called exercise. What does it do for you? When performed properly and in sufficient quantities, you will be able to move, feel, and look better, in that order. In general, as your fitness improves, you will be able to do more physically. When you do more physically, your health will start to improve and you will feel better. Finally, as your health improves, so will your appearance.

You know that you need and should exercise, but for one reason or another, you may not do enough of it, or do it effectively enough. To make things worse, when you stop exercising, your body gets weaker. This makes it physically harder to exercise, which in turn makes you less inclined to do so, mentally. This vicious cycle continues, and before you know it, you're out of shape and unhappy with the way you look, feel, and perform. People who try to catch up by exercising on the weekends when they're "free" often end up with so-called "weekend warrior" injuries. Even if you are motivated enough to actually start exercising, it is all too easy to get off track. Miss a workout here or there and before you know it, you're back to square one again. Most workouts take too much effort to become a habit. That's why many resolutions, New Year's or otherwise, usually fail. All of these issues make this problem so much harder to fix.

In this chapter, you will learn about the various aspects of fitness and how it affects your performance. The next two chapters will cover how exercise affects your health and appearance.

Fitness: What Does It Mean?

The word "fitness" is used frequently, but what does it really mean? One definition from the Oxford English Dictionary is "the condition of being physically fit and healthy." This doesn't tell us much, since we now need to define what it means to be "physically fit." A more useful definition from the same dictionary is "the quality of being suitable to fulfill a particular role or task," but it doesn't mention what those roles or tasks are. I interpret those as the things we need to do to get us through life. These include activities related to our job, grooming, obtaining and eating food, chores, recreation, and so on. Physical fitness is therefore how well you can move around and do the activities in your life. If you are physically fit, it is easy for you to take part in these physical activities. That means it doesn't take much effort for you to do the things you normally do throughout your day. In addition, you are able to engage in recreational or more intensive activities. If you are not physically fit, moving around is difficult and burdensome for you. Furthermore, you probably do not have enough reserves to participate in more intensive activities, even at a recreational level.

Now that we know what physical fitness means in general terms, we need to determine what exactly affects a person's fitness so we can improve it. Physical fitness is more than just strength or endurance. It is the combination of all the attributes that affect your ability to perform physically. These attributes include strength, power, flexibility, agility, endurance, balance, and coordination. A deficiency in any one of these will decrease your performance. Let's go over each attribute in detail and see how they affect physical performance.

Strength

Strength is the basis of all movement, and it affects many other components of fitness. It is simply the maximum amount of force you can exert at any particular point in time. The more weight you can support, the stronger you are. For example, you would need more strength to carry a 100 pound box of office equipment than a 50 pound box.

However, strength is used for more than just carrying things around. It is also particularly important in maintaining your posture. The muscles throughout your body, especially in the core, help keep your body in proper alignment. If they aren't strong enough to do so, your body will end up in unnatural positions, such as a slouch. Over time, this leads to pain in various parts of your body, especially the back. So, it is very important to make sure that you develop sufficient strength to maintain good posture.

Note that strength is a static measurement. It does not reflect how fast you can move an object, which is determined by your power. Strength and power often increase and decrease together, although not necessarily by the same amount. However, without sufficient strength, you cannot develop power.

Since power and several other fitness attributes are affected by strength, it makes sense to focus on it first. As your strength increases, it becomes easier to improve on the other attributes. Fortunately, you can increase this all-important attribute quite easily with consistent training. When you expose your muscles to incrementally heavier loads, your muscles adapt by growing stronger. This is the core principle behind all strength training programs.

Power

Power is a measure of dynamic strength. It determines how fast you can apply your strength. The more strength you can apply in a shorter amount of time, the more powerful you are, and the more explosive your movements will be. Power is important for many movements, such as sprinting, swinging a bat or racquet, jumping, punching and kicking, to name a few. For example, when trying to catch a bus, you'll need more power to run faster. The additional power pushes your body forward faster with each step. Similarly, the higher you want to jump, the more power you will need. The additional power enables you to push yourself off the ground faster, thereby overcoming gravity even more.

Your muscles contain two kinds of muscle fibers, fast-twitch and slow-twitch. Fast-twitch fibers are more effective at quick, intermittent contractions, while slow-twitch fibers are better at sustained contractions. To increase your power, it is important to develop your fast-twitch muscle fibers. This is best done by training with fast, explosive-type, dynamic movements.

Flexibility

Flexibility reflects the range of motion of your joints. Your overall flexibility is largely determined by the pliability of your muscles, since they are capable of the greatest change in length. The more flexible you are, the further you are able to move. This is a very important aspect of fitness. Flexibility not only enables you to do more, it also helps reduce your risk of injury during physical activity. For example, let's say you are walking to the grocery store when you step on a patch of ice. Your foot slips out from under you and you nearly land in a front split. If you are like most people who can't do splits, you will likely pull or tear a muscle from this accident because your legs muscles aren't able to stretch that far. However, if you are flexible enough, you will probably be fine.

It is important to note that flexibility and strength go hand-in-hand in protecting you from injury. Flexibility without strength is a recipe for injury. Without sufficient strength, flexibility can actually increase your risk of injury because you are not strong enough to protect your joints when they are moved to the limits of their range of motion. Therefore, it is very important to develop strength along with flexibility.

You can improve your flexibility in a number of ways. The most obvious one is static stretching. It is important to stretch properly and frequently. You want to make sure that you are stretching the muscles, not tendons or ligaments, which are not meant to stretch much. If you stretch incorrectly, you'll end up weakening your joint and perhaps even injure it. If you stretch intensely on one day, take it easy the next day so your body can recover. I recommend stretching lightly on these off days, just enough to loosen up. This way you don't become tight again from the previous day's stretching while still allowing your body to recover properly.

Agility

Agility is the ability to change your body position and direction effectively and efficiently. Obviously, agility is important for many sports, but it is also important in daily life. Let's say you are crossing the street when you see a distracted driver run a red light and head straight for you. If you are agile enough, you just might be able to dodge the car.

To improve your agility, you should train with complex movements that challenge it. Doing so will increase your awareness of your body, the signals it is giving you, your surroundings, and your ability to react appropriately. Since agility is a high-level attribute that depends on all of the other fitness attributes, it is important to train the other attributes first. This way, you will benefit more quickly when you work on agility-enhancing training exercises.

Endurance

Endurance is how long you can sustain an action or activity. For example, it affects how long you can play a sport. On a day-to-day level, it helps you get through a busy day at work or at home chasing a toddler around the house.

On a more basic level, muscle endurance is important in maintaining good posture, such as when sitting for long periods of time. Even if your muscles are strong enough to keep your body in the proper position at first, without enough endurance, they will get tired as you stay in the chair. Over time, you'll start slouching, which will cause all sorts of problems for your body.

Fortunately, endurance can be improved simply by doing the desired action or activity for incrementally longer periods. Over time, your body will adapt by improving its efficiency so that it can perform for longer.

Balance

Balance is the ability to sense and maintain the body in a stable position. This can be as simple as staying upright when standing, or as difficult as doing free-standing handstands or balancing on a tightrope. Balance depends not only on your senses, but also in the speed of your reflexes and the strength and power of the muscles reacting to restore stability.

For example, when you trip on an uneven sidewalk, a good sense of balance can help prevent you from falling. When your foot catches, your body pitches forward and starts falling. First, you have to react fast enough to re-adjust and plant your foot in time. Then, you need enough strength in your leg and core to catch your weight and keep you from falling any further. As you can see in this example, strength plays an important role as well.

A good sense of balance will also improve the efficiency of your movements, as well as your overall agility. You won't need to make as many corrections to your body position and you'll spend less effort maintaining your stability while moving. This enables you to perform even better.

Balance training is a great way to work on opposing muscle groups simultaneously while improving your ability to listen to your body. Since balance requires a feedback loop between what you sense and how you react, you'll learn to be more aware of the signals that your body parts send to your brain. At the same time, your muscles will keep making corrections to your body position. When a correction by one muscle is too big, the opposing muscle will kick in to counteract the overcorrection. This cycle goes on continuously and is what enables you to maintain your balance.

Coordination

Coordination refers to how well you can direct the various muscles in your body to produce the desired movement. A lack of coordination results in inefficient movement and in the worst case, puts you at risk of injury. Highly coordinated movement is efficient and reduces your risk of injury. Coordination also enhances your ability to perform complicated movements, which is critical to improving performance.

Even though each of us is born with different levels of coordination, it can be improved with practice. You just need to learn to listen to your body more closely and pay attention to how it actually reacts when you tell it to move. You may be surprised to find out at first that your body is not doing exactly what you intended or thought you were doing. Once you realize that, it is just a matter of refining the accuracy of your movements.

Improving Your Fitness

All of these attributes of physical fitness can be improved with exercise. They can also worsen if you don't do anything. The key to improving your fitness is consistency. It is more effective to take smaller actions on a regular basis than to take larger ones sporadically. You will not only make consistent progress, you will also be much less likely to get injured. Getting hurt can stop and even reverse your progress because you'll need to take a break to let the injury heal. The amount of progress lost depends on the duration of the break. However, you can't rush the healing process because you'll end up exacerbating the injury.

How fast an attribute improves depends on the type of exercise that you do. For example, weightlifting works largely on strength, power, and coordination, while long distance running works mostly on endurance and coordination. The exercises in the One Minute Workout work on strength, muscle endurance, flexibility, balance, coordination, and, to a certain extent, power. They will help improve your fitness so you can be more active physically.

⏱ 9

Improving Your Health Through Exercise

The most important thing I learned from being a physician is that your health is your most important asset. It is the great equalizer. I have seen patients from many walks of life. It doesn't matter how much money you have or how famous you are, without your health, you can and will lose everything. This unfortunate consequence is something I see repeatedly when taking care of patients at the end of their lives.

When I first started practicing medicine, I often counseled patients to exercise more. Like many other doctors, this usually meant telling them to get at least 30 minutes of exercise three times a week, and to be more active in general (taking the stairs, park farther away from the store, etc.). Generic advice, and perhaps some customized suggestions if they were receptive, was all I could give them. Many of my patients didn't have the time or money to go to the gym or take fitness classes. As a result, the effectiveness of the "diet and exercise" prescriptions was less than spectacular. However, after having used the One Minute Workout to transform my own body and the lives of those who have used it, I can see it as a simple but useful tool for people to help turn their health around. If you are a healthcare provider, I challenge you to suggest the One Minute Workout to your patients and see what happens. I think you will be pleasantly surprised.

Your doctor has probably told you that exercising is good for your health. But how does it improve your health, exactly? These days, there are tons of articles and stories out there about what's good and bad for your health. You hear about numbers like BMI, VO_2 max, HDL, LDL, waist-to-hip ratio, fasting glucose, systolic and diastolic blood pressure, and many others. You also hear about diseases and conditions such as Type 2 diabetes, hypertension (high blood pressure), obesity, hypercholesterolemia (high cholesterol levels), and so on. There is so much out there that you might be tempted to tune it all out and do nothing. But that is the biggest mistake you can make.

The truth is, it doesn't need to be all that complicated. Basically, your health reflects how well your body can do what it needs to do and also how well it can keep that going. Your body is affected by what you put in it (what you eat and drink) and what you do with it (your level of activity). If your body doesn't get enough of what it needs, you develop a deficiency that can lead to illness. On the other hand, if your body gets too much of what it needs, your systems get clogged up, which can also lead to illness. The key is to match the input with the output. This way, your body keeps humming along happily. All of the numbers mentioned earlier are different ways doctors and scientists estimate how well your body's systems are running. However, they are just that, estimates. You can't rely on just one measurement to determine if you are healthy or not. You must to look at multiple measurements and at the overall picture.

For example, body weight by itself does not accurately indicate your health status. You could be heavy because you are tall and muscular, or light because you are short and thin. Even the commonly used Body Mass Index (BMI), which is the ratio of your body weight to the square of your height, is not that accurate. It is fairly good for getting a quick ballpark estimate, but there are many false positives and negatives. For instance, very muscular people can have BMIs that put in them in the overweight range, while tall people with too much fat but little muscle can still be in the normal range. These incorrect categorizations occur because the mathematical formula does not account for the fact that muscle weighs more than fat.

Even though researchers are still looking for more accurate predictors of health, we know one thing: muscle is good for your health. So, instead of focusing on your body weight, you should be more concerned about having enough muscle and being healthy for your weight. This can be achieved by improving your body composition, which means finding a healthy ratio between your body fat and muscle. For most people, this involves building more muscle, whether they are overweight or underweight.

Why is Muscle so Important?

Muscle is important because it does so many things for the body. First of all, it is more metabolically active than fat tissue. At rest, a pound of muscle burns about six calories a day, while a pound of fat burns about two calories a day. That's three times more calories burned without doing anything!

Now, you might say, "If I added ten pounds of muscle, that's only 60 more calories per day." Keep in mind, however, that while the absolute number of calories burned by muscle at rest may not seem like that much more, it isn't negligible. Over time, these extra burned calories add up. At 60 calories a day, that adds up to six pounds of fat a year!

But wait, there's more. Muscle can do something else that fat can't— move your body around. That means the additional muscle uses up even more calories as they help you move around. Plus, don't forget that the more muscle you have, the easier it is to move. The easier it is to move, the more likely you are to move. Increasing your physical activity boosts the number of calories burned by your muscles.

Furthermore, some of your muscle fibers naturally break down when you use them, such as during exercise. Your body responds by repairing those fibers, making them stronger, so that they can handle similar stresses in the future. This repair process consumes calories and continues even after you stop exercising, contributing to what is sometimes called the "afterburn effect." The more intensely you use your muscles, the more fibers need repair, and the greater the number of calories burned to fuel the repair process. All of this means that having more muscle increases your ability to burn more calories faster.

However, the importance of muscle goes beyond burning more calories. Muscles also protect your joints by providing support. If you don't have enough muscle to provide sufficient support, you will develop poor posture, which leads to more muscle and joint pain. In fact, this is an exceedingly common cause of back pain.

Additionally, muscles act as shock absorbers during impact activities. For example, when you run, your heel hits the ground repeatedly. This shock travels up your lower leg to your knee. If you have enough upper leg muscle, you can reduce the shock to your knee by bending it more and absorbing some of the impact energy into your muscles. On the other hand, without sufficient muscle, more of the shock necessarily needs to be absorbed by other tissues in the joint, such as the cartilage and ligaments. This translates into more wear and tear on the tissues that don't regenerate like muscle can. Over time, this wear and tear adds up, until eventually something gives out and you end up with a serious injury.

Recent research has even shown that muscle mass can be a good predictor of how long you may live. A study of 3,659 men 55 years or older and women 65 years or older published from the University of California, Los Angeles in 2014 found that having more muscle mass was associated with a lower risk of death in this group of people.[1] While more research still needs to be done, this finding certainly suggests that maximizing and maintaining muscle mass is a good idea.

Exercise and Specific Health Conditions

As you can see, your weight and BMI are not the deciding factors for your health. Building more muscle will help your body metabolize more energy so that it is easier to lose excess fat. It will also help protect your joints from the stress of carrying your weight. Most importantly, the ability to be more active will improve your health in a multitude of ways, some of which we'll go over below.

Hypertension (High Blood Pressure)

Your blood pressure depends on several factors, such as blood volume, the pumping strength of your heart, and the elasticity or springiness of your blood vessels. Your blood vessels actually have muscles in their walls that help maintain their elasticity. This elasticity improves blood flow and helps even out highs and lows in blood pressure. Just like other muscles, if you don't use them, you lose them. When those mus-

[1] Preethi Srikanthan, Arun S. Karlamangla, "Muscle Mass Index as a Predictor of Longevity in Older-Adults," *The American Journal of Medicine*, 2014, 127(6), 547-553.

cles shrivel up, blood vessels become weak and stiff. Without sufficient elasticity, your body increases blood pressure in order to get blood to flow to the rest of the body. Chronic high blood pressure means your heart has to work harder, which can lead to heart failure. It also damages other organs, such as your kidneys, and leads to organ failure over time.

Exercise temporarily increases your blood flow and pressure. This gives the muscles in your blood vessels a workout so they can continue to work properly and keep your blood pressure normal. Since the heart and blood vessels are connected to each other in the cardiovascular system, exercise also gives your heart a workout, so that it, too, can continue to function properly. This is one way to conceptualize how exercise helps keep your blood pressure in a healthy range and prevents hypertension.

Obesity

To put it in simple terms, obesity is the result of your *mind* being unable to manage your energy appropriately. Why? Because the state of your body is a result of your behaviors over time, and your mind controls your behaviors, such as what you eat and when you move. This may sound harsh, but reality is quite stark. I went through a period of denial myself before waking up to reality and realizing that I was the one responsible for gaining so much weight.

Regardless of what kind of metabolism your body has, you need to match your energy input with your output, or else you will have an energy imbalance. Your energy comes from food, and it is either used up through activity and bodily functions, or it is stored as fat. If you keep taking in less energy than you need, your body starts burning stored fat to make up for the energy deficit. However, as you burn off fat, your body's energy needs also decrease. So, in order to keep losing fat, you will have to cut down on your energy intake even more. This is why you reach a plateau in your weight loss efforts even if you religiously stick with the same diet plan.

Exercise is a way to raise your energy output and burn fat calories. As you lose fat, your body's energy requirements will decrease and you will need to exercise even more to keep losing weight. This is a reason many people reach a weight loss plateau despite regular exercise. However, if you exercise intensely enough for your body to be stimulated to repair and build new muscle, your body will continue to burn more energy even after that particular exercise session. The gained muscle will further increase your body's energy requirements so that your energy balance will tip in the negative direction. This is one way you can make it easier for your body to manage energy better.

Fortunately, obesity is a very curable problem and exercise is one half of the solution. The other half is eating appropriately for your body's needs. By adjusting your inputs and outputs properly, you can reverse obesity and the health problems associated with it. Furthermore, you can prevent the development of a more serious medical condition called Type 2 diabetes.

Type 2 Diabetes

Type 2 diabetes is a condition where your *body* is no longer able to manage energy properly, and it is often a result of a prolonged period of obesity. Specifically, it is a problem with your body's ability to produce and respond to insulin. As a result, your body can no longer maintain blood sugar levels within normal limits. Over time, high blood sugar levels lead to a slew of other medical complications, such as cardiovascular disease, strokes, kidney failure, retinal damage, and neuropathy, among others. Fortunately, Type 2 diabetes is preventable and even curable in the early stages.

Your body has a complex system for managing energy. It figures out what to do with the energy from the food you eat and how to provide energy for physical activity and bodily functions. It also manages how energy stores are shifted from one type to another. As long as you match your energy intake and output reasonably closely, all of this happens in the background. You don't even need to think about it.

When your body functions normally, your body can also handle energy imbalances for short periods of time fairly well. These imbalances can be small, such as getting a second helping or skipping a meal one day. They can even be as extreme as starvation and feasts for short periods of time, such as a few days. However, when these imbalances persist chronically, such as during obesity, your body's energy management system starts breaking down. This is when you develop Type 2 diabetes.

Once you have Type 2 diabetes, many other parts of your body also start having problems due to chronically elevated levels of blood sugar. First, the smallest blood vessels in your body become damaged, resulting in reduced blood flow to the areas they serve. As this continues, other organs and body systems start taking damage, such as your kidneys, brain, heart, eyes, and nerves. Your kidneys stop functioning, so you need dialysis. Your heart can't get enough oxygen, and you start having heart attacks. Your brain gets small strokes all over the place, killing tons of brain cells, and your mental abilities along with them. Your eyes go blind and your nerves feel like they are on fire, before they stop working completely. Even parts of your body start rotting off, because they don't receive enough blood. I have seen countless patients with Type 2 diabetes, many with these complications. It is truly a devastating and gruesome disease to have.

While you can take medications such as insulin to help your body manage energy better, they will not cure you of the disease. At best, they will delay the onset of the above-mentioned complications. Medications are not curative because there is still an underlying energy imbalance beyond what your body can handle on its own. However, if you fix the energy imbalance early enough, you can actually reverse some of the effects of Type 2 diabetes. This can be accomplished by eating appropriately and doing exercises that improve your body composition. I have seen patients do this and get off of diabetes medications, including insulin, and essentially cure themselves of their disease.

Exercise and Osteoporosis

Despite advances in medical treatments, complications from osteoporosis, a significant loss of bone density, are still quite common. Effective treatment of osteoporosis requires more than just medication. You also need to get enough usable calcium through your diet. Just as importantly, you need to do exercises that stress your bones, so that they use the calcium to grow stronger. This means lifting things, whether they are weights at the gym or bags of groceries. Walking on the treadmill does not help. Besides increasing bone density, these weight-bearing exercises also strengthen your muscles. When you gain strength, you are able to move better, maintain your balance better, and reduce the risk of falls and injuries. This is another way that exercise combats the potentially devastating complications of osteoporosis.

Slowing Down the Aging Process

While the fountain of youth has yet to be discovered, exercise can slow down certain effects of aging. For example, we all start losing muscle mass after a certain age. For men, this starts at about age 32. As you lose muscle mass, you lose strength, and with it, your ability to move around. Have you ever noticed that many elderly people tend to have more difficulty moving? This is because they lost too much muscle to move well anymore. The good news is that this muscle loss is easily countered by doing exercises that maintain, or even build, muscle. I am always amazed by my elderly patients who look and move around like a person 10 to 20 years younger than their actual age. When I ask them how they do it, the answer is invariably the same—they exercised and stayed active their entire lives.

Reducing Pain

Pain is one way our body tells us something is wrong. When a muscle or joint hurts, pain discourages us from using it so it has a chance to heal. However, sometimes the pain becomes chronic, and we stop using the affected body part for long periods of time. As a result, the muscles in that area become weaker as they atrophy, and other muscles need to kick in to compensate. The problem is that now these other muscles have to work harder, sometimes to the point of injury. In addition, even if the original injury heals, the weakened muscles may continue to get weaker because you have become accustomed to using other muscles to compensate. This results in a vicious cycle of pain and injury that continues indefinitely unless there is focused intervention.

To break this vicious cycle, the weakened muscles need to be strengthened, so that they can do their job effectively. Once this is achieved, the compensating muscles can go back to normal work loads. This helps restore normal function and reduces, or even eliminates, the pain.

Another way to look at our bodies is to compare them to a concrete building. Our muscles are like the concrete, while our bones are like the metal frame. The building is not meant to be held up by just the frame and rebar, but together with the concrete. When the concrete is broken, the frame is exposed to increased stresses and becomes damaged. Similarly, our bodies are not held up just by bones. They are also supported by our muscles. Without sufficient strength in the muscles, our bones and joints are exposed to more wear and tear and eventually become damaged.

Even though the cartilage in our joints acts as a shock absorber, it gets damaged and worn out. This leads to osteoarthritis and joint pain. Your joints will last a lot longer if you take care to protect them. One way to do this is to strengthen the muscles that stabilize and support your joints. This reduces the likelihood of moving your joints in unintended ways and injuring them. Furthermore, the shock-absorbing capabilities of strong supporting muscles can prolong the useful life of the cartilage in your joints.

Now, let's talk about back pain. It is commonly the result of weakness in the core muscles. Without sufficient core strength keeping the bones in your spine aligned, they fall out of position. On the outside, all you see is poor posture. However, on the inside, it is much worse. Nerves get pinched and the cartilage discs in your spine get squished in unnatural directions. Once damaged, cartilage essentially never heals, because it doesn't have a blood supply. Without healthy cartilage, bones start rubbing against each other, and bone spurs might grow, leading to even more irritation and pain. These joint and nerve pains exist on top of any muscular pains that develop due to strength imbalances. Fortunately, if you start improving your core strength and posture before these injuries become permanent, your back pain can be resolved. Even if the pain has become chronic, it can still be improved. My mother has had severe back pain for over 30 years. Through those years, she sought treatment from a variety of physicians, chiropractors, acupuncturists, and Chinese herbalists, among others, without much success. However, once she started doing One Minute Workout exercises regularly to strengthen her muscles, her symptoms improved dramatically.

Sitting: A Silent Killer

A big motivator for me to create the One Minute Workout was to wage war on sitting. Sitting is killing us and we don't even know it. In this day and age, many of us spend most of our waking hours sitting down. We sit many hours at work, and when we come home, we sit down for several more hours in front of the computer, television, phone, or tablet. With so much time spent sitting, it's no wonder we don't get much exercise. However, it's not just the lack of exercise that is dangerous. The act of sitting itself can also be dangerous to your health, especially if done for prolonged periods of time. In fact, recent research studies have correlated long periods of sitting with a 40% increase of death from all causes.[2] Even worse, this risk is NOT reduced by exercising regularly a few times a week.

While the exact mechanisms of how sitting causes harm to our bodies haven't been completely established yet, we know a few things. First of all, when you sit, your metabolism changes and you burn fewer calories than when standing or moving. Combined with a tendency to eat too many calories, this is obviously undesirable. To make things worse, sitting also reduces your body's ability to break up and burn fat. Not only are you burning fewer calories overall, it also takes longer to burn off any fat calories.

Second, sitting for prolonged periods affects your ability to move. You already know that you can develop pain from sitting too long, and pain makes it hard to move. However, staying in one position for too long can also cause your muscles to shorten, thereby decreasing your flexibility. The less flexible you are, the harder it is to move, and you become more prone to injury. In extreme cases, you can even develop

---

[2] Hidde P. van der Ploeg et al., "Sitting Time and All-Cause Mortality Risk in 222,497 Australian Adults," *Archives of Internal Medicine*, 2012, 172(6), 494-500.

contractures, something that you usually see in people who can't move on their own and don't receive physical therapy.

Finally, sitting for long periods of time decreases blood circulation. This allows blood to pool in your body, especially in the legs and feet. Is this dangerous? You bet. When blood pools, it tends to clot. When clots form in your leg veins, your legs swell and hurt. In medicine, we call these clots Deep Vein Thromboses, or DVTs. While they can be quite painful, the real danger is when a clot breaks away and travels to your lungs, causing a blockage called a pulmonary embolism that kills off part of your lungs. In extreme cases, these clots can actually stop blood from being pumped by the heart, causing instant death. This is so dangerous that doctors routinely give hospital patients prophylactic blood thinning injections to reduce the risk of these clots from forming. Fortunately, if you are healthy, you won't need these injections, but you do need to watch how long you sit at a time. Even healthy people can get these dangerous DVTs.

Now that you know how dangerous sitting can be, what can you do? The best thing to do is break up long periods of sitting by getting up and moving around. During these breaks, take a walk, stretch, or even better, kick your metabolism up a notch by doing some exercises, such as one from the One Minute Workout. This will help protect you from the dangers of prolonged sitting, plus you'll feel better and be more productive.

* * * * * * * *

The key points to remember are that muscle provides strength, strength is the basis for all movement, and movement is essential to health. We are not meant to be sedentary beings. The more we move, the more likely we are to be even more active, which helps promote health. In addition, physical activity and focused intervention can help correct imbalances and accelerate recovery from injuries. You don't have to go overboard and go run a marathon right away. Just take steps each day to be more active, and you will be surprised by how much better you feel.

How Exercise Makes You Look Better

Let's face it, we all care about the way we look. Even if your primary reason for exercising is to improve your health, I'm sure you wouldn't mind if you looked better as well. Unfortunately, there are many exercise myths out there that don't do much for getting results. One thing is for sure, though—there is no magic bullet that will make you look great quickly *and* keep it that way. Successfully enhancing your appearance requires knowing what works and what doesn't. It will also require making some changes in your life, and enough time for those changes to take effect. However, it is definitely possible, no matter what you look like now.

The Three Components of Body Shape

Your body shape is determined by three major components: skeleton, muscles, and fat. Your skeleton is the frame for your body shape and it determines overall aspects such as your height, shoulder and hip width, and limb length. Once you are fully grown, you can't do much to change your bone structure, outside of surgery.

Your muscles are attached to your skeleton and enable you to move. They round out the bony outline of your skeleton by adding smooth curves to your frame. Each muscle can change in size and shape, depending on how it is used or not used. So, you can change the look of a body part to a certain extent by working on the appropriate muscles. Similarly, you will lose a desired shape if you don't maintain the muscles providing that shape.

The body fat right under your skin covers up your muscles and smoothes out your body shape even further. As you gain fat, it will start hiding the outlines of the individual muscles and their striations, making your body shape more uniform. If you have too much body fat, it will cover up all of your muscle definition and start hanging from your frame. This leads to common "trouble" areas such as underarm flab (a.k.a. "teacher flab"), belly flab, and love handles, among many others. The generally undesirable "potbelly" look is a result of the fat around your internal organs, also known as visceral fat, building up to the point that it pushes the abdominal wall outward.

In general, fat is gained and lost in a fairly uniform manner. Therefore, you can't lose fat in just one part of your body to make it look thinner or more defined. However, the good news is that when you lose enough fat, the effects will show throughout your entire body, making you look better everywhere.

Changing Your Body Shape

Now that you know how your body shape is determined, let's look at ways to change it, along with some common questions and myths. Based on our discussion above, the two components of body shape that you can change are the amount of muscle and the amount of fat that you have.

Let's talk about changing fat first. To gain fat, all you have to do is eat more calories than your body can use. The excess energy will be converted to fat and stored throughout your body for future use. Losing fat seems like it should be as simple as eating fewer calories than your body needs. However, losing fat is the opposite of what your body wants to do. Therefore, it takes significant effort and willpower on your part to do this.

To increase muscle mass, you will need to train your muscles by pushing them to their limits. In contrast, losing muscle mass doesn't require much work. All you have to do is not use your muscles. Your body will automatically break down any muscle tissue that has not been used in a while. This can happen amazingly quickly, in as little as a day or two of bed rest. Fortunately, with the One Minute Workout, you can maintain the muscle you already have without spending much time.

Which is Better: Losing Fat or Building Muscle?

To bulk up, you will need to build muscle mass. Bigger muscles will fill out your frame and provide more pronounced contours. However, it is just as important if you are trying to trim up, or increase definition and tone. The bigger and more distinct your muscles are, the more they will show through the skin and fat covering them. If your muscles are small, then your fat will play a much bigger role in determining your body shape. This means you'll have to work even harder to lose more fat just to tone up your body.

If you only focus on fat loss efforts, you will inevitably lose muscle mass at the same time, which is counterproductive. When you lose muscle mass, you'll have to lose even more fat for your underlying body shape to show. Even worse, having less muscle mass makes it more difficult to burn excess fat. To top it off, you end up weaker and less physically fit. All of this makes it that much harder to achieve the look that you are aiming for.

The bottom line is that you should always be building muscle, or at least maintaining what you have. Muscle makes it easier to shape your body and it also makes it easier to lose fat. In addition, it will help improve your health.

Doesn't Unused Muscle Transform into Fat?

Contrary to common belief, unused muscle does not turn into fat. When it is broken down, the basic building blocks your muscles are made of are recycled for use elsewhere in the body. The fat comes in when you keep eating the same way you did when you had more muscle. When you use your muscles less than before, the decrease in physical activity means you burn fewer calories. Also, when your body breaks down unused muscle tissue, your baseline energy requirements go down. If you eat the same amount as you did before your muscle mass decreased, you will have an energy surplus. Your body stores this extra energy as fat.

This is why it is easy to become fat and flabby even if you had a lot of muscle at one point. This is a common mistake many people make when they become less active. To prevent this from happening, you will have to decrease the amount you eat appropriately. I made this exact mistake when I stopped exercising due to long hours at work. Despite the decreased activity and lost muscle mass, I kept eating the same amount I was used to eating. All of this extra energy was packed on each day as fat. Once I realized what was happening, I started eating smaller amounts appropriate for my new body composition and activity level. This small change in my habits stabilized my body weight and stopped fat accumulation.

Won't Strength Training Make Me Big and Bulky?

Many women focus only on fat loss efforts and shun muscle building exercises when trying to improve their body shape. The fear is that they will develop big, bulky muscles like bodybuilders. However, this fear is completely unfounded. Unless you make a dedicated effort to build big bodybuilder-like muscles, your muscles won't look like that. Just ask anybody who is seriously looking to bulk up. You'll find that they put in a lot more effort and dedication than a basic fitness workout. Rest assured that the exercises in the One Minute Workout will help you develop a lean, athletic build.

Can't I Just "Spot" Fat Burn?

As mentioned earlier, your body fat increases or decreases in all parts of the body at the same time. For example, you cannot "burn" fat away from just your abs, or just your triceps. But, you can train the muscles in these areas so that they become big enough to provide the desired shape and definition. In fact, unless the fat layer is excessively thick, you can make your muscles big enough so that they show through the fat. This happened to me after I started working out with the One Minute Workout. The exercises built up my core muscles so much that my abs started showing through the belly fat that had accumulated over the years. The "one-pack" became a "two-pack," then a "four-pack," then finally a "six-pack." This all happened without any special fat loss efforts.

Low Intensity or High Intensity?

You may already know that working out at different intensities burns energy at different rates. The harder you work out, the more calories you burn in the same amount of time. What you may not know is that your body uses different fuel types depending on the workout intensity. When performing lower intensity "cardio" type exercises, you burn a larger proportion of fat fuel than carbohydrate fuel. This is why the fitness industry has misleadingly dubbed this intensity range as the "fat-burning" zone. The higher the intensity, the greater the proportion of carb fuel is used. So, based on this, it would be natural to assume that doing more low intensity cardio exercises will burn more fat calories, but this would be a mistake.

It all comes down to some simple math. The problem is whether you want a bigger slice of a small pie or a smaller slice of a bigger pie. Let's say you walk on a flat treadmill for 30 minutes at a leisurely pace and burn about 200 calories. If 80 percent of those calories were from fat, you would burn a total of 160 fat calories. Now, let's say you go twice as fast on the treadmill with a 15 percent incline for the same amount of time. You would then burn about 580 calories. Even if you burn only 40 percent fat at this higher intensity, you would still burn over 230 fat calories. That's almost one and a half times the fat calories burned for the same amount of time! Plus, don't forget that you've also burned an additional 310 carb calories.

But we're not finished yet. After you work out, your body needs to replenish its energy stores. Any carbs you eat post-workout first go to replenish the carb stores, then the excess gets converted to fat. That means the fat calories you just burned can come right back.

For example, let's say you do a low intensity workout like a slow jog or walk. You've burned some fat calories, and now it's time to eat. Since, you've burned mostly fat, your carb stores are still mostly full. So most of the carbs that you eat are converted straight to fat, undoing much of your workout efforts. You could choose to eat fats instead, but those calories get stored as fat as well. And, don't forget that fat contains more than twice the energy of carbs, so you'll also have to eat a lot less.

On the other hand, if you do a higher-intensity workout like running or riding a bike at a brisk pace, your body burns more fat *and* carb calories. This time, the carbs in your post-workout meal will go toward replenishing your carb stores first. Much less of them, if any, will be converted straight to fat. That means more of the fat calories you burned away during the workout stay gone.

This is a major reason people can do low-intensity cardio workouts for months or years and still look the same. Higher-intensity exercises are more effective and will get you the most results for time spent. In addition to cardiovascular benefits, you will burn more fat calories, be able to eat more carbs, and stimulate your muscles to grow, thereby initiating the "afterburn effect."

Now, I'm not saying low-intensity exercise won't change the way you look, just that it will take longer. In fact, my dad had a sizable potbelly for many years. Then one day, he got a new job that required him to take two trains, transfer to a bus, then walk rapidly for another thirty minutes just to get to the office. Walking an hour each day to and from the office burned away his sizable potbelly in about a year, without any changes to his diet. It was amazing. Unfortunately, the potbelly came back when he changed jobs again and no longer walked as much. If you don't have an hour to walk every day and a year to wait, then your best bet is to increase the intensity of your workouts.

Section III

Your Mind and Body

⏱ 11
Staying on Course

The truth is, most workout systems will work … if you can stick with them. But that's the biggest problem. Does the following sound familiar: You hear about a new workout program from a friend or a TV commercial and think "This is it! This is how I'm going to get in shape!" Then you try it out and realize it's harder than you thought. You might do it a few more times, or even for a few more weeks and then you stop. If you had gained any benefits (e.g. weight loss, more muscles), they eventually disappear because you aren't able to keep up with the workout.

I ran into the same problem over and over again with many other workouts. Whether I tried going to the gym, exercising outdoors, or doing workout videos at home, in the end, I couldn't stick with them. That's why I designed the One Minute Workout to especially address these issues. What makes this system different? It was designed based on understanding how we make decisions, and how those decisions become lasting behaviors and habits. This makes it easy to get started, and even easier to keep going. And in the event you get off track, getting back on track is as effortless as getting started the first time.

To make a truly lasting improvement in your life, you need to change your habits. Most of us have bad habits that we want to change into good ones. Unfortunately, changing a habit can be really hard. I want to share with you some ways to make forming good habits easier. Once you learn these methods, you will be better-equipped to make any type of change you want in your life.

Setting Goals and Objectives

One of the keys to being successful is setting goals and objectives. Without these, you don't know where you're headed. If you don't know where you're headed, you'll never know if you're making any progress, or if you are even going in the right direction.

First, let's talk about goals versus objectives. While they may seem similar, objectives and goals are quite different. Goals are general directions or intentions that you work toward. They are usually broad in scope and have long or unspecified time frames. On the other hand, objectives are much more specific. They include concrete details and operate on a shorter time frame. Most importantly, they are measurable. For example, losing weight is a goal. On the other hand, saying you want to lose ten pounds in six weeks is an objective that moves you in the direction of your goal.

When you decide to make a change in your life, you are setting a goal. To improve your chances of success, take some time to write down objectives that will help you achieve the goal. By writing them down, you help yourself remember them over time, and you become accountable to yourself. Include as much detail as you can think of. Then, set a timeline with specific dates by which you want to achieve your objectives. This way you'll know whether what you are doing is working or not, and if you are making progress fast enough.

When you set a lofty goal, it may seem out of reach, especially in the beginning. Unfortunately, this is where many people quit. In order to achieve something big, it is even more critical to set smaller, more reachable objectives that will pave the way. These smaller objectives form a road map for you to follow so you don't get lost along the way. More importantly, they keep you motivated. It is easy to become discouraged when you are working toward a far-away goal. Smaller but more frequent victories over intermediate objectives are great for reaffirming that you are on the right path.

Keeping Track of Progress

Keeping track of your progress is extremely important, but many people don't do it. While tracking may seem like an extra step to take, it provides several benefits. First, it can keep you motivated. Each time you update your log, you can see your efforts accumulating, so any improvements that you have made will be apparent. You will take pride in all that you have accomplished, and this will keep you wanting to do more.

Second, the act of writing down your progress will make you more accountable. When you update your log regularly, it becomes obvious when you start slacking off. For example, if you stop working out, a quick look at your log will tell you exactly how much time you took off. This can give you a kick in the butt and get you back on track. Without a log, it's easy to think that your previous workout wasn't that long ago, so you're more likely to put off working out to another day. What ends up happening is that your workout gets pushed back further and further until you completely forget about it.

Finally, keeping a written log means you don't have to keep track of all the details in your head. An easy-to-reference log tells you if you are behind schedule, and exactly where you left off earlier. This makes it very easy to get back into the workout groove and maximize your time and effort.

Re-evaluating and Readjusting

Setting out-of-reach goals and repeatedly failing to reach them is a sure way to become discouraged. However, this doesn't mean you shouldn't set big goals. It just means that you may need to readjust them from time to time, whether it's the details of a particular objective, or the time frame for reaching it. This is the same principle that you should take with anything in life, whether it's your career goals, a hobby project, or a relationship.

When you first set a goal, you don't necessarily know all the details about it, nor exactly how to achieve it. As you work your way toward it, you accumulate information and experience that can help you evaluate your goal and objectives better. Armed with this information, you can determine if the original details are still realistic or not. If not, you are now better informed and can make more realistic adjustments.

Each time you reach an objective, take a step back and look at what you have achieved and where you should go next. If you decide that the original goal is not obtainable, you will still have achieved your smaller objectives. Reflecting on them will show you what you have gained and that your efforts were not in vain.

Setting Goals with the One Minute Workout

By choosing to do the One Minute Workout, you probably already have some goals in mind. They could be general, like improving your health, or more specific, like increasing your strength or building more muscle. Whatever they are, write them down. Next, write down some specific objectives to create your roadmap. For example, if you are new to working out, you might aim to do your first pull-up within six months. You would then set smaller objectives to help you do that, such as mastering a 135° Bent Arm Hang in one month and starting an Eye-Level Bent Arm Hang by three months. If you are already in shape and looking for a challenge, you can set harder objectives, such as doing a Full Planche in a year. For this example, you could set intermediate objectives such as mastering the Frog Stand in one month and mastering the Tuck Planche in three months.

With these smaller objectives in place, just keep track of your progress each time you work out. Each time you do an exercise session, write down how many seconds you performed the exercise. Organize your log so that you can easily see how many sessions it takes for you to finish your minute each day.

As you build your exercise log, you'll know if you're on track or not. For example, let's say that by the end of the first month, you are already working on the Advanced Frog Stand, which is harder than the Frog Stand. This means you are a bit ahead of schedule and you can continue working out as planned. On the other hand, if you are still struggling to master the Frog Stand at this point, then you are behind schedule. That means you need to take another look at what you are doing to see what needs to be changed. Perhaps you aren't working out frequently enough, or maybe you are working out too much and not giving your body enough time to repair itself. It may even be something other than your workout, such as nutrition. Make sure that you are eating well enough, so your body has enough nutrition to repair and strengthen your muscles. Also, make sure that you aren't doing things to sabotage your body and progress, such as drinking alcohol excessively or smoking. Once you identify what is holding back your progress, you'll be able to make the appropriate changes. However, if you can't find anything that is holding you back, then you may need to adjust the time frame for the objective.

Making and Changing Your Behaviors

Now that you know how to set goals and objectives, you'll need to make sure that you take actions that keep you moving toward them. Below, we'll take a look at why we take certain actions and not others. We will also go over some ways that you can keep yourself on track. Understanding yourself better will help you change your habits more naturally.

Whether you actually end up taking a particular action or not is determined by three factors: motivation, difficulty, and a trigger. First, you need to have sufficient motivation to do it. How much motivation you need depends on the second factor, which is how difficult it is to do. If something is easy to do, you don't need to be very motivated to do it. On the other end of the spectrum, it takes way more motivation to do something that takes a great deal of effort. The additional motivation is what drives you to spend the extra effort. Finally, you need a trigger to remind you to take the action. Without the trigger, you can still fail to perform an action even if the other two factors are sufficient.

Let's look at a few examples to illustrate the importance of these factors.

Motivation vs. Difficulty of Action (Ability)

Let's say you're a little hungry and want a snack. You happen to have a bag of chips. It's pretty darn easy to open up the bag and start snacking, so you do so. Action completed. In this example, opening up the bag of chips and eating it is virtually effortless. Therefore, you only needed a small amount of motivation (being a little hungry) to take the action.

What if you didn't have any snack-like foods around the house? You'd have to leave the house and go to a store or a restaurant to get something to eat. Now, if you were just slightly hungry and therefore not really motivated, you might just say "forget it" and wait until the next meal. In this case, the action of snacking is not taken. But, if you were starving and therefore really motivated, you might run out to the store and get your favorite chips, probably along with a bunch of other bad food choices. In this example, you can see that it takes more motivation to complete an action that requires more effort.

Now let's use a similar example to show why you might choose a less healthy action over a healthier action. Let's say you're hungry and you want a snack. You have a bag of chips right on the counter and an orange in the refrigerator. You could easily open the bag of chips and eat the conveniently bite-sized pieces of crunchy tastiness to satisfy your hunger. Or, you could go to the fridge, wash off the orange, peel it, then separate it piece by piece before eating it. Which would you rather do? Unless you had a strong motivation to eat the orange, you would probably eat the chips since it takes less effort.

This example illustrates why it is so easy to make poor health decisions. In general, humans are lazy, and snack food companies know this. Junk food brands also make their products addictively tasty, so that once you start eating them, it is hard to stop. However, you can overcome this by making it easier for you to take healthy actions. For example, you could store the unhealthy snacks out of sight, where they are harder to reach, while placing the healthier options out in plain view. You could even go further and prepare the healthier options ahead of time, so that eating them is essentially effortless.

But what if you're motivated enough to do something, but you still keep forgetting to do it for one reason or another? For example, you make a New Year's resolution to get in shape and even get a home gym, but you still don't exercise. This is where the third factor comes into play.

Enter the "Trigger"

A trigger is something that causes you to take action. Some are motivational, some make things easier, and some are just reminders. When you have sufficient motivation for an action, a trigger is all it takes to make you do it. However, without the necessary motivation for the difficulty level, the trigger won't work.

Going back to the last example, creating a trigger of some sort would make you take action. For example, you could set an alarm to go off as a reminder to exercise, or you could put the home gym somewhere you pass by frequently during the day. When you see it, you will be reminded to exercise. In this case, a neutral trigger is all it takes to make you take action.

However, triggers can also make you take one action over another. Imagine you are watching television and you are hungry. You want a snack. You have a bag of chips on the counter and an orange in the fridge. You are about to get up to grab the chips when a commercial for a new diet comes on. You see the before and after pictures and think to yourself, "I should really watch my weight!" So you end up going to the fridge and getting the fruit instead. Here, the diet commercial was a trigger that made you take an action that you otherwise would not have taken. In this case, a trigger helped you make a healthier decision.

Now, we'll look at another example about working out. Let's say someone, who we'll call Bob, has been in excellent shape for his whole life, and he loves working out. He is super-motivated to work out. Even though his gym is an hour away, his workout takes two hours, and it makes him sweat like crazy, he still does it. Despite the tremendous amount of effort it takes to work out, his high level of motivation drives him to do it anyway.

But what if you are not like Bob? If you are like most people, you are in average shape or worse. You know you should exercise (average or low motivation) but the gym is too far away, and you are so "busy" that you don't have even an hour to spend on the actual workout. It takes too much effort for your level of motivation, so you don't work out. As you get more out of shape, working out takes even more effort and you become even less inclined to do so. As you can see, this quickly becomes a vicious cycle. Before you know it, your motivation falls off the charts and your physical ability to work out declines so much that it is almost physically impossible for you to do any exercise. Even a strong trigger, such as hearing news of your best friend having a heart attack, doesn't get you working out, because it is just too hard for you now. While this may seem like an extreme example, it is unfortunately true for too many people.

How can we change this? The less motivation you have, the easier we need to make it to take action. So, what if you bought some workout videos, or a treadmill for home? Chances are you would be excited about it for a short while, but then reality would catch up to you. It still takes a lot of time to work out, even though you are doing it at home. Plus, you still get sweaty, and who wants to be all sweaty? Before you know it, the treadmill becomes another clothes rack and the workout videos sit in the corner collecting dust. Now, if you happen to hear that your best friend just had a heart attack, you might be inclined to dust off the videos and start working out for a while. But as time passes and the news becomes distant, you'll probably let the workout videos collect dust again. Taking this example to the extreme, you might argue that if your best friend had a heart attack every month, you would keep dusting off the videos and keep working out. However, if that were the case, your best friend wouldn't be alive very long, right? So, in the end you still wouldn't be exercising.

* * * * * * * *

In order to make permanent changes to your body and health, you need to create changes in your behavior that last. Because the One Minute Workout System is as short and convenient as possible, it requires less motivation to exercise on a regular basis. This is critical, since your motivation level will vary quite a bit. It will change throughout the day depending on your mood and your schedule. It will also change over time as your original inspiration becomes more distant, and other sources of inspiration or distraction pop up.

In addition to minimizing the motivation threshold necessary to exercise, the One Minute Workout System works extremely well with reminder systems. A reminder notification can trigger you to perform a short exercise session. In fact, that is what I use myself. The online virtual trainer sends me workout reminders on my phone and tells me what exercise to do. It also keeps track of my exercise sessions and progress all in one place. You can check it out for yourself at www. OneMinWorkout.com.

Further Reading

As I was developing the One Minute Workout, I figured out the three factors on my own through trial and error and my past experiences. Later, when I showed a friend my workout system, he mentioned the work of Dr. BJ Fogg, the director of the Persuasive Technology Lab at Stanford. It was amazing how well my system fit the behavioral model he proposed. Some time later, I was fortunate enough to hear him speak at a conference, and let me tell you, his work is quite inspiring. To learn more about his behavioral model, visit his website at bjfogg.com.

⏱ 12
What Should I Eat?

The goal of the One Minute Workout System is to make you healthier and to help you achieve your goals more easily. Physical activity is only half of the solution. Eating well is the other half. While there isn't a rigid diet that you need to follow, there are general guidelines. These guidelines will help you make sustainable changes that will enable you to reach and maintain your goals. I'll also clarify some misconceptions about food and share some tips that have helped me. When followed in conjunction with the One Minute Workout, your gains will be realized more quickly.

General Guidelines

Make Small Changes

Don't make drastic changes right away, such as cutting out all carbs, eating only 500 calories a day, or never eating your favorite foods again. If you do, you risk stressing your body and mind too much. Both will miss what they are used to and you will suffer from cravings. The excessive stress can also be counterproductive, causing your body to react in the opposite way to what you want. Plus, each time you slip up, which you will likely do at some point, you will beat yourself up over it. Eventually, this will make you give up and go back to your old habits.

Instead, make small changes that you almost don't notice. For example, eat one less slice of pizza at a meal, add one more piece of fruit every other day, or take the stairs instead of the elevator once a day. This gives your body time to physically adjust to the changes in your behavior, and your mind to become used to the changes in your body. Once that change becomes your new norm, you can make further changes. Using this step-by-step method, you can achieve and sustain even the most extreme changes with relative ease.

Change One Thing at a Time

Just like making big changes right away, making too many changes at once, even if they are small, will over-stress your body and mind. Start with one change and let yourself get used to it. When that has become your new norm, you can make another change. Use this technique to achieve and maintain changes in several different aspects of your life.

Don't Deprive Yourself

If you really like eating something, don't cut it out of your diet completely. If you do, you'll end up feeling guilty every time you crave it. Your cravings will also become stronger and more frequent until you finally give in and pig out. Instead, just reduce the amount that you eat, whether in portion size or the number of times you eat it. This way, you won't feel guilty eating it, and since you aren't depriving yourself, your cravings will be less intense. Follow this and you will have greater ability to control when and how much of your treats you eat.

Don't Starve Yourself

Similarly, don't try starving yourself by skipping meals entirely in an attempt to lose weight. Doing so will actually do more harm than good over time. Without the necessary nutrition, your body can't defend and repair itself properly. This increases your risk of injury and illness. Furthermore, your body will also break down your muscles for energy in response to starvation. In extreme situations, prolonged starvation can lead to serious medical conditions, such as heart failure and severe electrolyte imbalances.

Starving yourself is also mentally unsustainable. You will just feel bad all the time, and your mood will be affected. This can spill over into other aspects of your life, such as work productivity and relationships with people. This mental stress is compounded with the physical stress that your body faces from starvation. Too much stress of either kind is unhealthy.

To make this worse, when you finally stop starving yourself, your body will soak up whatever you eat in order to replenish the energy and nutrition stores that were depleted during starvation. Going back to your usual diet before starving won't keep the weight off, since your body will return to the steady-state weight it was before the starvation period. More often than not, you will end up overeating and gain just as much weight as you lost, if not more. Starvation is counterproductive, potentially dangerous to your health, and makes it more difficult to reach your weight loss goals.

Don't Work Out on an Empty Tank

Working out on an empty tank is even worse than starving yourself. The effects of starvation are magnified when you exercise on a stomach that has been empty for a while, such as in the morning before your first meal. At this point, your energy stores are low, and there is nothing in your stomach to replenish them with. Let's say that you decide to hop on the treadmill to burn some calories in the morning before breakfast. You figure that since you haven't eaten anything yet, you can start the day with a calorie deficit. However, your body requires two different kinds of fuel during exercise: carbohydrates and fats. Even if you are doing low intensity "fat burning" cardio, your body still needs carbohydrates for energy. Since you haven't eaten breakfast yet, your body is essentially running close to empty. Therefore, it starts cannibalizing your muscle proteins and converting them into the needed energy. In the end, you don't lose any more fat than usual, BUT you lose valuable muscle.

So, if starving and working out on an empty tank is bad, what can you do? The key is to have just enough carbohydrate energy on board to last through the workout. This way, your muscles don't get broken down for energy, and you won't have excess carb energy on board that will be converted to fat later on. Furthermore, the fat that you burn off during the workout will stay off. Of course, you will still need to keep working on your muscles to maintain them.

Out of Sight, Out of Mind

Many of our eating vices are based on impulse decisions. When you see something you like, you remember or imagine how good it feels to eat it. The visceral imagery is so enticing that you usually end up eating it. To prevent this from happening as frequently, keep the foods you are trying to cut down on out of sight. If you don't see it, you won't think about it. This means you will be less inclined to eat it. Try putting the foods you are avoiding in a drawer or cabinet that you don't open frequently. The refrigerator is not a good place to hide foods because we often rummage through it when we are looking for things to eat. However, if it needs to be refrigerated, stick it in the back where you can't readily see it.

This is exactly what I did when I wanted to cut down on junk food. When I used to leave opened bags of chips on the counter, I found that I could go through a large bag in a few hours by myself. Every time I took a little break and wandered into the kitchen, I would see the bag and eat a few chips. However, after putting the chips back in the cabinet each time, I ate them less frequently. Now, a bag easily lasts a week or more.

Drink More Water

Water makes up the majority of our bodies and it is crucial for our bodies to function properly. Water is not only critical for the function of your cells and body systems, it is also one of the major ways wastes and toxins are removed from your body. That being said, many of us don't get enough water each day. You can consume water in a variety of ways, including soups, juices, and other beverages. However, if you are watching your waistline, then plain water is the best choice. That's what I ended up doing when I was trying to lose weight. I used to drink juice and juice-based drinks all the time. When I cut out the juice drinks that contained high fructose corn syrup, I stopped getting heavier. When I went a step further and replaced most of my fruit juice intake with plain water, I dropped several pounds. If you do the math, it makes a lot of sense. At about 110 calories per eight-ounce glass of juice, replacing five glasses of juice with water meant I cut out 550 calories a day!

You can lose even more weight by drinking water to reduce snacking. Sometimes you want to eat because you are just a little hungry but it isn't quite meal time yet. When this happens, you can cut down on unhealthy snacking by drinking a glass of water. It will fill your stomach up for a short time, which can be just enough to tide you over until the next meal. It can also help you eat less during the meal, thus further reducing your caloric intake. This is a great way to get in the recommended eight glasses of fluid per day.

Now, you might ask "Do we really need eight glasses of water per day?" Yes and no. You lose water every day through both sensible losses, such as going to the bathroom and sweating, and insensible losses, such as water vapor escaping when you breathe. To replenish these losses, you need to consume water, whether it is in the form of plain water, beverages, or moisture found in foods such as fruits, vegetables, and meats. You don't necessarily need to drink an additional eight glasses of plain water each day. Just make sure you get enough fluids to keep your body well-hydrated. So yes, you do need a good amount of fluid each day, but not all of it needs to come from drinking plain water.

Is eight glasses of fluid right for everyone? To explain, I'll have to show you some calculations. While this recommendation is quite popular, it is likely meant for the "typical" patient as used in medicine, which is a 70 kilogram man. When a patient can't eat or drink, doctors need to maintain the patient's hydration. Fluids are administered intravenously and the amount given is estimated as follows:

$$4 \text{ mL/hr/kg for the first 10 kg } +$$
$$2 \text{ mL/hr/kg for the next 10 kg } +$$
$$1 \text{ mL/hr/kg for the remainder of the weight}$$

So, for a 70 kg man, this would be 110 mL/hr:

$$10 \text{ kg} \times 4 \text{ mL/hr/kg } +$$
$$10 \text{kg} \times 2 \text{ mL/hr/kg } +$$
$$50 \text{ kg} \times 1 \text{ mL/hr/kg}$$
$$= 110 \text{ mL/hr}$$

Over 24 hours, this person would receive 2.64 liters of fluid which is about eleven 8-ounce glasses of fluid. Keep in mind, if you are eating, you'll get a few glasses of water through your solid food and the rest through drinking. So, for the "typical" 70 kg male, the eight glasses of fluid recommendation is reasonable. You would need more if you are heavier and less if you are lighter. With that being said, this recommendation should only be used as a rough guideline. How much fluid you actually need will also depend on your particular body and state of health, how active you are, and what kind of foods you eat.

Can you drink too much water? It is possible, but really difficult. There is a medical condition called psychogenic polydipsia where a person is driven to drink very large quantities of water, on the order of gallons a day. The amount of water is so large that the electrolytes in the body are thrown out of balance and other physiologic processes are disrupted. However, if you are healthy and you eat a balanced diet, your body should be able to handle as much water as you can *comfortably* drink.

Forgive Yourself and Give Your Body a Chance to Recover

If you have a big or heavy meal one day, don't beat yourself up over it. Your body is surprisingly good at accommodating fluctuations, and it will return to baseline if you give it a chance. Just take it easy the next day or two and eat smaller amounts of lighter food. This will give your body time to clean out the extra calories, salt, and other overloaded nutrients. In a few days, you should be back to the way you were before the big meal. If you don't give your body time to clean out, the extra nutrients will start accumulating in your body, leading to conditions like obesity and hypertension.

Mix It Up

Don't eat the same thing every day. Instead, mix it up. Besides keeping food interesting, this reduces the accumulation of unhealthy substances in your body. If you keep eating the same thing every day, you may be ingesting small amounts of toxins, natural or otherwise, which are found in that particular food. Normally, your body will try to get rid of these toxins. However, if the same kinds of toxins keep coming in every day, your body's cleansing ability may be overwhelmed. Regularly changing what you eat helps prevent this from happening and gives your body a chance to remove these toxins.

Reaching Specific Goals

Now that we have some basic guidelines, let's look at some examples to see how you can use them to achieve specific goals with less effort.

How Do I Eat Fewer Calories?

If you are overweight, then it shouldn't be surprising that you may be eating too much. But, it doesn't have to be hard to eat less. You just have to go about it in a sustainable way. Your stomach is used to being stretched to a certain size at each meal, and unless you fill it up, you'll just want to eat more. So, don't cut your portion size in half or skip meals. If you do, you'll just end up feeling hungry and unsatisfied all the time. Plus, it will be really hard to resist snacking frequently between meals.

Instead, decrease your portion sizes by just a little bit every few days or so. Put one less item on your plate, or take a smaller serving of whatever you are eating. Each small change will be much less noticeable to you, and it will give your stomach a chance to get used to being stretched less from the meals. Over time, this series of changes will add up and be quite significant. You might even end up wondering how you ever ate so much before.

So, the next time you order pizza, eat just half a slice less. If you really feel that you need a little more to fill you up, drink some water or grab a small piece of fruit. After doing this the next few times you order pizza, try cutting out another half slice. Before you know it, you'll be eating significantly fewer calories and still feel full.

Also, to help you feel more full throughout the day, you can also try eating more protein earlier in the day. Replace some of the carbs in your breakfast and lunch with protein so you don't add on additional calories to those meals. Besides keeping you feeling full longer, you'll also have more protein available to help repair and build muscle.

How Do I Eat More Fresh Fruits and Vegetables?

You already know that fresh fruits and vegetables are good for you. However, you don't need to cut out your favorite foods and eat like a rabbit to be healthier. Find some fresh fruit or vegetable that you like, or can at least tolerate, and add a bit of it to one of your meals in the day. Can't do that every day? Try doing it one or two days a week at first. When that becomes a habit, go up from there.

For example, you decide you want to eat more apples because they are crisp and delicious, plus you heard they keep the doctor away. You start out by eating an apple on one day as a snack. Take the next day or two off from apples and then it's another apple day. After doing this for a week or two, you start eating apples (or some other fruit—remember, it's best to mix it up!) on most days and only take one day off each week. Keep making these small changes, and eventually, you'll be eating a piece of fruit every day. You might even find that you'll want to explore other kinds of fruit and vegetables!

If you like fruit smoothies, you can also consider getting a blender and keeping a variety of fruits available in the fridge. To make it easier, pre-wash your fruits, so making the smoothie is as easy as possible. You can even add some vegetables into the smoothie such as carrots, cabbage, kale, and spinach. Just add a small handful or a few small pieces so your blender still runs smoothly. This will also keep the flavor from changing too much. If you are worried about cost, you can get uglier or riper (but sweeter) fruits that are on clearance. You won't care about looks when it's going into the blender!

How Do I Eat Less Carbohydrates?

Carbohydrates have gotten a bad rap recently, but they really aren't bad for you. In fact, they are a great and necessary source of energy. However, since foods packed with carbs are cheaper and easier to get these days, it's really easy to eat too much of them. That is the real reason to watch out for carbs.

So, the next time you eat something packed with carbs, don't freak out and swear it off. Just follow the guidelines outlined earlier in this chapter about eating less. Try eating half of whatever you're eating and save the other half for later. Or try replacing it with a protein-rich food that will make you feel full with the same number or fewer calories.

How Do I Drink Fewer Sugary Drinks?

While there's nothing wrong with enjoying sugar-laden drinks like soda once in a while, it becomes a problem when you drink them all the time. The extra calories are literally poured into your system. To put the brakes on this deluge of liquid calories, start out by replacing just one of your drinks with water each day. As you get used to it, replace more of your drinks with water. Before you know it, you'll be drinking more water than any other beverage.

I know this method works because I used to be someone who hated drinking plain water. It was too bland. But, I wanted to lose weight, so I started replacing one of my meal-time drinks with water each day. Since I was drinking the water with a meal, the lack of taste didn't bother me as much. This way, I didn't completely deprive myself of fruit juices, which I preferred. Eventually, I was surprised to find that I started enjoying the "taste" of water, especially refreshingly cold, filtered water right out of the refrigerator. There was something about the crisp coldness and clean feeling of the water after drinking it that was really appealing, so I started replacing other drinks with it. Over time, I cut out several hundred calories a day using this method.

How Do I Eat Less Junk Food?

We all know we should eat less junk food … but it just tastes so good! That shouldn't be a surprise, though. These easy-to-eat snack foods are specially engineered (yes, engineered!) to taste good, and to keep us eating more. Unfortunately, they are usually packed with things that we want to eat less of, such as salt, carbs, and fats. So how do you cut down on the amount of junk food you eat? Again, make small changes that you won't really notice.

Just like cutting down on sugary drinks, you can replace the junk food during one snacking session with something healthier. Instead of eating chips and cheese curls several times a day, grab an apple, an orange, or some other fruit or vegetable one of the times. You might be surprised by how much better you feel afterward. You will also feel fuller and end up consuming fewer calories.

It also helps to wash out the junk food taste that lingers in your mouth afterward. This aftertaste often makes you want to keep eating more, even after you have closed the bag of chips and put it away. Try eating a few bites of a crunchy fruit or vegetable after eating junk food. Apples, carrots, and other crunchy fruits and vegetables work well, since they help clean the junk food off of your teeth and cut through the flavoring. You can also try drinking some water if you don't have some fruit or vegetables handy. Once the aftertaste is gone, you will be less likely to crave more of the junk food.

Finally, don't go shopping at the grocery store when you are hungry. You'll be more likely to pick up unhealthy snack foods and other poor food choices. If you have to go when you're hungry, make a list of things to get beforehand and stick to the list as you pick out items. This way, you'll be less likely to buy the foods you are trying avoid.

How Do I Eat Less Salt?

If you didn't already know, we tend to eat too much salt these days. Not only is all of this extra salt bad for your blood pressure and cardiovascular health, it makes you gain weight by retaining water. This extra water is necessary to balance out the extra salt so that your body systems can continue working properly. Even if you do nothing else differently except eat less salt, you will lose a few pounds. This happens because the additional water weight goes away as your body gets rid of the extra salt and adjusts to the smaller load of daily salt it has to handle.

The first step in eating less salt is to know where it's hidden. We get a lot of it from processed foods like canned goods, fast food, frozen meals, and restaurant food. A good amount of salt is also hidden in breads, bagels, and similar baked goods. Read nutrition labels and look for how much *sodium* the food contains. This way, you get an idea of how much salt you get with each serving. Don't get tricked by tiny serving sizes on the labels. If you eat the entire can of soup, find out how much salt is in the entire can, not just one serving. You'll be surprised how much salt you are actually eating. Once you know where your salt is coming from, you can apply the guidelines from this chapter to reduce the amount you eat.

To Supplement or Not to Supplement

I found that if you are aiming to maintain or build muscle at a normal pace, there is no need to use protein or vitamin supplements. Just make sure you eat a balanced diet as well as some protein close to the time you work out. The protein can be in any form, such as meat, eggs, fish, tofu, dairy, etc. This way, your body has the raw materials it needs to repair itself at the most critical time, right after exercise. If you are spacing out your One Minute Workout sessions throughout the day, snack on some protein throughout the day, or try to get some protein in with each meal. This will help you build dense, lean muscles without gaining much weight. The average person simply aiming to be healthy and fit doesn't need to worry about taking protein supplements like whey powders.

However, if you are trying to bulk up or gain strength rapidly, then you may need to use protein supplements. Follow the instructions for the supplement you use and be sure to maintain a well-balanced diet. Drink plenty of water to help your body wash out the metabolic waste that comes from working out hard. To ensure you get the most out of your workout and supplements, make sure you also get enough vitamins and micro-nutrients for your body to repair itself and build mass efficiently. Help your body process energy well by getting enough of the water-soluble vitamin B family. Don't forget that your muscles are only as strong as the tendons they are attached to, so make sure you get enough vitamin C, which will help your body produce the collagen crucial for healthy ligaments and tendons. Finally, be sure to get enough calcium and vitamin D so that you have strong bones for your muscles to act on.

What About Exercise Drinks?

For the vast majority of people, there is no need to use exercise drinks such as Gatorade®, Powerade®, and other similar products when working out. These products often advertise their ability to replace electrolytes lost from exercise. However, what they really offer is hydration and some energy, usually in the form of carbs. Even though these exercise drinks do contain some electrolytes, you are unlikely to run into an electrolyte deficit during the average workout. In general, you need to work out long and hard for several hours (e.g. running a marathon) in order for you to sweat out enough electrolytes for this to be the case.

For most people, staying hydrated while exercising should be the main concern. Drinking water is the simplest way to do this. If you prefer flavored drinks, you can try adding a small piece of cut fruit to your water, such as a slice of orange, lemon, or strawberry. Although I recommend water that you flavor naturally yourself, there are a variety of pre-flavored waters available that you can try. Unless you need the extra sugar, look for brands that have zero or few calories, and preferably no artificial sweeteners.

Exercise drinks are designed to contain a source of energy, usually sugar, so you have fuel to continue working out. The problem is, if your workout isn't long enough to deplete your carb fuel stores, this extra energy isn't going to help you. If you're looking to burn calories, gulping down a bottle of your favorite exercise drink will basically negate a portion of the workout you just did.

On the other hand, if you train really hard and deplete your energy stores, then an exercise drink would be a quick way to replenish them. Without sufficient energy for the workout, your body will go into a catabolic state where it starts converting your muscle mass into energy. This is obviously counterproductive and it can set you back significantly. I've had personal experiences with this in the past where I went on long bike rides without enough food on hand. Aside from making the rides miserable, I found that my strength levels dropped significantly afterward, setting me back about two weeks of workout progress. Needless to say, I am not keen on making that mistake again.

* * * * * * *

The key to success in changing and maintaining your diet is to make one small change at a time. Resist the urge to change too many things at once. Be sure to give yourself time to adjust to each change. As these changes add up, you will start seeing significant improvements in your body. Most importantly, you will have a much easier time maintaining the changes because they will have become the new norm for you. And remember, whatever your goals are, always do your best to eat healthily and drink plenty of fluids.

⏱ 13

Getting to Know
Your Muscles

In this chapter, I will introduce your muscles so that you have a better understanding of how your body moves. This will help you target your areas of focus with appropriate exercises. If you are already familiar with this material, feel free to skip this chapter.

Understanding how your body moves is an important part of both exercise and daily life. Knowing which muscles enable each movement empowers you to move more safely and effectively. You will know if you are doing the exercises correctly and whether you are targeting the proper muscles. Furthermore, you will be able to plan your workouts better to achieve your goals faster. Finally, when you look in the mirror, you will know whether you have achieved what you expected from your hard work.

My anatomy class in medical school opened my eyes to how complex movements can be. Even though a single muscle produces a specific movement in a joint, the movements we make as a whole can involve a multitude of muscle groups. I learned how many of our muscles can act in more than one direction. Along with pulling and pushing, muscles can also create concurrent twisting movements. Working together with the large muscles are a myriad of smaller and less well-known muscles throughout the body that contribute greatly to our movements.

Since there is enough information on anatomy to fill volumes, this chapter will just be a superficial introduction to your muscles. The anatomical images in this chapter are from the 20th edition of Henry Gray's *Anatomy of the Human Body*. If you would like further detail or additional anatomy images, you can refer to textbooks such as Frank Netter's *Atlas of Human Anatomy* or search online.

Below, we will go over the major muscle groups, the movements they help produce, and bit about their appearance. In Sections IV and V of this book, each exercise entry includes a muscle map that indicates which muscle groups are targeted by that exercise. Be sure to take a look at it before doing the exercise so that you know which muscle groups you should pay attention to.

Upper Torso

Pectorals ("Pecs")

The pectorals cover a large part of your upper chest. There are actually two different sets of pectoral muscles—the *pectoral major* and *pectoral minor*. The *pectoral major* is the bigger of the two and lies over the smaller *pectoral minor* muscle. These prominent muscles are often considered a visual indicator of a person's overall strength, although it is not always accurate. They act on the upper arms in several ways, including pulling them toward the middle of the body, pulling them forward, and also rotating them toward the middle of the body. Since the pectorals act in so many directions, they are active in many arm pushing movements and are very important for shoulder joint stabilization. A classic exercise that trains these muscles is the pectoral fly.

Serratus Anterior

The *serratus anterior* muscles are arranged in a layer on the sides of the rib cage. Since they are thin and flat, they are usually not very visible. However, when they become large enough, you can see them just below the pectorals, right where you would normally see ribs. They act on the shoulder blades by pulling them forward into a protracted position. This action helps stabilize the shoulder blades during movements that involve the shoulder joints. Punching is a classic movement that engages the *serratus anterior*.

Trapezius ("Traps")

These huge fan-shaped muscles are located on the upper back and neck. They help raise your shoulders, pull your shoulder blades together, and pull the shoulder blades down. They are used in both pulling and pushing movements and also provide stabilization for the shoulders, back, and neck. Movements in different directions develop different parts of the large trapezius muscles. Therefore, make sure you work on a variety of exercises to ensure even development.

Rhomboids

The rhomboids are upper back muscles located between the shoulder blades in the layer behind the trapezius. These often-neglected muscles play an important role in many upper body movements, since they stabilize the shoulder blades. They accomplish this by pulling your shoulder blades towards each other, such as when you squeeze them together.

Latissimus Dorsi ("Lats")

In Latin, the word *latissimus* means "broadest," and *dorsi* means "back." These muscles are in fact the broadest muscles in the back. They start at the shoulder, extend downward along the back of the ribs, and end in the small of the back. They help pull your arms behind you and also toward the middle of the body. The lats work in conjunction with the biceps when you pull objects toward yourself, or pull yourself toward something, as during a pull-up or rowing movement. Well-developed lats contribute aesthetically by making your back look broader.

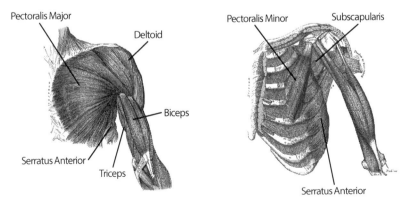

Left: Front view of superficial upper torso muscles.
Right: Front view of deeper upper torso muscles.

Arms

Deltoids

The deltoids are located on the outermost part your shoulders and help you move your arms forward, backward, and out to the side. They generally work with other muscles that stabilize the shoulder joint. When the deltoids get large enough, they develop into an oblong ball-like shape. In terms of aesthetics, they help define the groove between themselves and the biceps on the anterior (front) part of the upper arm. Similarly, they help define the groove between themselves and the triceps on the posterior (back) part of the arm. This area is one of the aesthetic trouble spots people are often concerned about. The lack of definition and the presence of dreaded "teacher flab" is usually due to excess fat and lack of muscle size in this area. Toning up the deltoids and triceps will do wonders for the area's appearance.

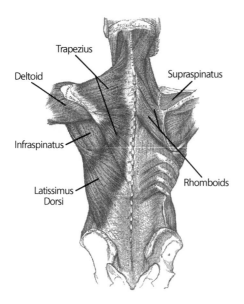

Left Half: Superficial muscles of the back.

Right Half: Deeper muscles of the back.

Rotator Cuff

The shoulder is a ball-and-socket joint, which allows for tremendous flexibility. However, that also means that it is one of the most inherently unstable joints in the body. Stability is largely imparted by the muscles that act on this joint. One of these major muscle groups is the rotator cuff.

This muscle group actually consists of four muscles. You can use the acronym SITS to remember them, which stands for the *supraspinatus*, *infraspinatus*, *teres minor*, and *subscapularis* muscles. This muscle group assists in many arm movements while simultaneously stabilizing the shoulder joint. Injuries to the rotator cuff are quite common, so it is a good idea to make sure to keep it as strong as possible. Strengthening the rotator cuff not only reduces the risk of future injury, it can also reduce pain from previous shoulder injuries.

Biceps

The biceps are located on the front of the upper arm. They help stabilize and bend your elbow joints. The biceps on each arm actually consist of two separate muscle "heads," thus "*bi*-ceps," which means "two headed" in Latin. These two muscles come together into a single end point near the elbow. They are used in many arm pulling movements, such as rowing and dumbbell curls. Like the pectorals, they are usually considered a visual indicator of a person's overall strength. However, upper body pulling movements involve other muscles, such as those in the upper back, so it is just as important to develop those muscles.

Triceps

The triceps are located on the back of the upper arm and help straighten and stabilize your elbow joint. This muscle's name comes from its three separate muscle "heads," which can be easily seen when well-developed. They are used in many arm pushing movements, like push-ups, pushing objects, and opening doors. Arguably, triceps are functionally more important in life than biceps. Well-defined triceps muscles can contribute greatly to your overall body aesthetics without making you look big and bulky. Toning your triceps, along with your deltoids, will also help improve the appearance of the underarm area.

Forearm Muscles

There are an astonishing number of muscles that control the movements of your wrist, hand, and fingers. Interestingly, most of these muscles have their bellies in the forearm, despite controlling relatively far-away joints, such as those in your fingers. They act on their target joints through an assortment of long tendons, sheaths and other soft tissues that help transmit and redirect their contractile strength. This arrangement enables your hand to be surprisingly strong, yet compact and agile. There are quite a few muscles, so I will only refer to them by functional group.

Wrist Flexors

The wrist flexors are located in the front of your forearm and help you bend your wrist in the direction of the palm.

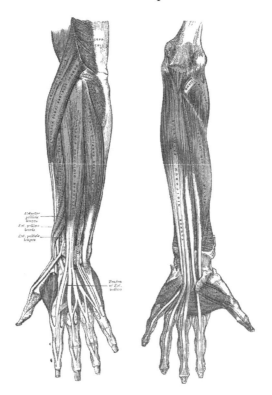

Left: Wrist and finger extensors.
Right: Wrist and finger flexors (grip muscles).

Wrist Extensors

The wrist extensors are located on the back of your forearm and help you bend your wrist in the direction of the back of your hand.

Grip Muscles

The grip muscles are also located in your forearm and help you close your fingers so that you can maintain a grip on whatever you are holding.

Core

You hear a lot about core strength these days, but do you know why? Your core muscles perform at least two essential roles. First of all, they help your body maintain good posture, whether you are standing or sitting. Your core muscles help maintain the alignment of your vertebrae and natural curvature of the spine. One simple way to visualize it is to think of your spine as a radio tower and the core muscles as the guy-wires. The core muscles work together and pull in different directions to keep your spine upright. If one of the guy-wires is loose, the radio tower falls over. The same thing happens with your spine.

Good posture is important for maintaining a healthy back and reducing back-related problems, especially from prolonged periods of sitting. Sitting down puts your spine in an unnatural shape. Over time, the stress of this unnatural shape starts causing pain. That's why you may find your back hurting after sitting for extended periods of time. On the other hand, your spine is in its natural shape when you stand. Therefore, your back can often tolerate longer periods of standing. Without strong core muscles, your posture deteriorates even faster and your body is essentially crushed under its own weight, causing a static injury. Since so many people have weak core muscles, it is no wonder that so many people develop back pain.

Second, your core connects your upper body and lower body so that they can work together. Your body functions like the links in a chain. One link acts on the next one, which acts on the next one, and so on and so forth. The core is one of the links in the chain, and it is responsible for transmitting power from one part of the body to the other. As you know, a chain is only as strong as its weakest link. If your core is weak, it will not be able to transmit power effectively, and your performance will suffer. Even worse, your core muscles and spine can get injured when handling loads beyond what they can safely tolerate, such as when you are trying to lift a heavy box. These kinds of dynamic injuries are also extremely common causes of back pain. Instead of allowing your core to be the weakest link in the chain, you should make it the strongest. This way, it can handle whatever stresses are thrown its way. In addition to improved performance, you will lower your risk of injury and pain.

Lower Back (lower Erector Spinae)

The *erector spinae* consists of a multitude of muscle bundles that run along the spine. This group of muscles helps stabilize and move the

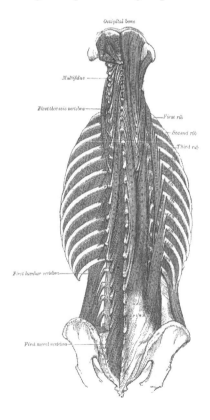

View of the deep muscles of the back, including the Erector Spinae. Note the multitude of long band-like muscles connecting various parts of the spine.

spine. The lower part of this muscle group acts on the lower back and is considered part of the core muscles. Strong lower back muscles will help improve your posture and aid in many dynamic movements. Weak lower back muscles are a common cause of lower back pain and are a common factor in back injuries. Unfortunately, our increasingly sedentary lifestyle contributes to the weakening of our lower backs, making back pain and injuries even more prevalent.

Abdominals ("Abs")

The *rectus abdominis* muscles are located on the front of the belly. There are actually eight parts to this muscle group, not six. The bottom two are located just below the navel and are harder to see, since there is usually more fat covering them than the upper abdominal muscles.

The abs are considered part of the core muscles and are tremendously important in a variety of movements. They are also extremely critical in maintaining good posture. Weak abdominal muscles can force other muscles to compensate, which can lead to pain and injury. While it is a good idea to work on the abdominal muscles frequently, make sure you do so while working on your lower back muscles. This will help ensure that the two are developed evenly, thereby reducing your risk of developing injuries and other problems due to muscle imbalances.

In order for the "six-pack" or "eight-pack" to be visible, you will need to have a relatively low amount of belly fat covering these muscles. The

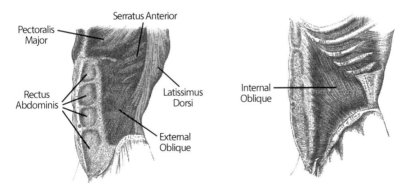

Left: Superficial muscles of lower torso.
Right: Deeper muscles of lower torso.

less belly fat you have, the more visible your six-pack will be. However, the bigger those muscles are, the more fat you can have and still see your six-pack. So, don't despair if you have trouble losing all of your belly fat, because six-pack abs are still possible!

Obliques

The oblique muscles are located on the sides of your abdomen and help bend and twist your trunk side-to-side. They are also considered part of the core muscles. They are often hidden under belly fat on the sides called "love handles." However, just like the abs, the bigger and stronger they are, the easier it is to see them. Unfortunately, these important muscles are commonly overlooked in many workouts.

Extended Core

With so much focus on core muscles these days, many of the nearby muscles are overlooked and under-trained. I call these the "extended core" muscles because they are the next link in your body's power chain. Most of the extended core consists of the various hip muscles. A weak extended core will also prevent effective transmission of power to the rest of the body, since it is now the weakest link. Make sure you work on the extended core muscles as much as the core muscles themselves.

Hip Flexors

The hip flexor group consists of several muscles around the hip joint that raise your thigh up, such as during a knee raise. The major muscles include the *psoas* and *iliacus*, but muscles from other groups also assist in hip flexion. The hip flexors play an important role in transferring mechanical forces through the hip joint. Since these muscles do not readily contribute to body aesthetics, they tend to be overlooked in traditional workouts. However, we will target them in the One Minute Workout. Weakness in the hip flexors can cause a variety of problems in walking, running, and many other activities.

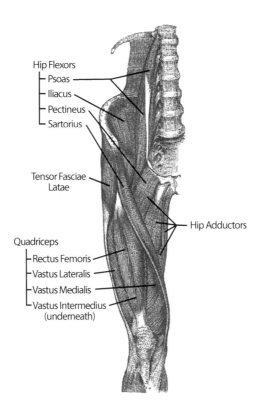

Front cut-away view of pelvis and upper leg.

Gluteus Maximus ("Glutes")

The *gluteus maximus* is the largest muscle in the buttocks region. It determines the overall shape of the butt, so if you want a good-looking butt, you need to work on this muscle. Mechanically, it plays a large role in extending your legs backward at the hip, and maintaining your posture in the standing position. Similar to the hip flexors, the glutes play an important role in transferring mechanical forces through the hip. Since many of us sit for long periods of time, this muscle tends to be weaker than it should be, which is why it is even more important to strengthen it.

Hip Adductors

The hip adductor muscle group pulls your legs toward your midline (aD-duction), enabling you to do things like squeezing your legs together. Hip adductors play an important role in maintaining side-to-side balance, as well as power transmission. They also help stabilize your lower body when you lift heavy objects.

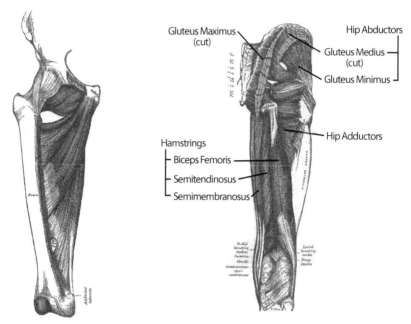

Left: Isolated view of major hip adductor muscles.
Right: Posterior view of pelvis and upper leg.

Hip Abductors

The hip abductor muscle group pulls your legs away from your midline (aB-duction), allowing you to move your legs out to the side. Some of the major muscles in this group include the *gluteus medius*, *gluteus minimus*, and the *tensor fasciae latae*. Since several of these muscles are located in the butt, developing this muscle group can help improve the shape of your butt by rounding it out. Similar to the hip adductors, they play an important role in maintaining side-to-side balance as well as power transmission.

Legs

Quadriceps Femoris ("Quads")

The large quadriceps muscles are located on the front of the thighs. They enable you to straighten your knee and help stabilize the joint. To a lesser extent, they also work with the hip flexors to help you bend your leg forward at the hip. The *quadriceps femoris* actually consists of four muscles (hence "quads"): *rectus femoris, vastus medialis, vastus intermedius,* and *vastus lateralis.* Strong quads are important in maintaining knee joint health and reducing the risk of injury. They should be trained as much as the hamstrings, which are on the backs of the thighs, so that they are similar in strength. Otherwise, the imbalance in muscle strength around the joint can contribute to knee injuries.

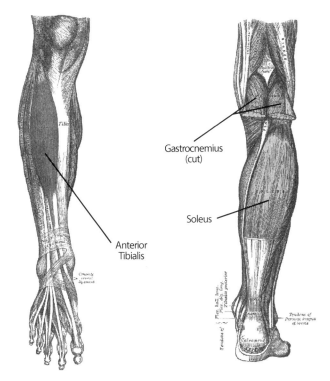

Gastrocnemius
(cut)

Soleus

Anterior
Tibialis

Left: Front view of lower leg.
Right: Posterior cut-away view of lower leg showing deeper muscles.

Hamstrings

The hamstring muscles are located on the back of the thighs. They enable you to bend your knee, as in a leg curl, and also help stabilize the joint. They also help extend your leg backward at the hip joint. This muscle group consists of three muscles: *semitendinosus, semimembranosus*, and *biceps femoris*. Strong hamstrings are important in maintaining knee joint health and reducing the risk of injury. As mentioned previously, these should be trained in concert with the quads to provide balanced strength and support to the knee joint. Flexibility in the hamstrings is also important for preventing injury.

Anterior Tibialis

The *anterior tibialis* muscles are located to the front and outside of the lower leg, right next to your shin bones. Their primary function is to bend your ankle up so that your toes don't hit the ground when you walk. They work with the other muscles in your leg to help maintain your balance.

Gastrocnemius and Soleus ("Calf")

The *gastrocnemius* and *soleus* are your calf muscles, located on the back of your lower leg. The *gastrocnemius*, which is easily visible, lays on top of the *soleus*. Together, they help you extend your ankle so that you can stand on tip-toe. You use them whenever you toe off during walking, running, and jumping. They also help absorb part of the impact from landing on your feet, thus reducing the shock to your ankles and knees. They also work with the other muscles in the lower leg to help maintain your balance.

Fixing Your Body

Many common joint injuries are the result of muscle weaknesses and imbalances. Shoulders, knees, back, ankles, elbows, you name it. However, you don't have to spend a lot of time or effort doing dedicated exercises to strengthen them. One Minute Workout exercises are designed to help strengthen the muscles associated with common joint problems. This system will also hone your body awareness and muscle sense, also known as proprioception. By doing these exercises, you will learn more about how to use your body and muscles appropriately. Ideally, you will also learn how to listen to your body better. All of this will help reduce the chances of injuring your joints.

When something goes wrong with our bodies, we tend to look for quick fixes. For example, if you hurt your shoulder doing yard work, it's easy to take a few pain pills to get you through the next few days. However, a "band-aid" solution isn't going to prevent it from happening again. The injury was likely caused by an underlying issue, such as poor technique or weak rotator cuff muscles. Unless the underlying problem is taken care of, you will likely injure your shoulder again. Eventually, it will become a chronic injury that may require more drastic treatments, such as surgery.

Below, we will go over some common joint problems and the exercise progressions that will help strengthen the muscles protecting those joints. If you have a particular area or problem you would like to address, just look for the name of the body part to find suggestions. I have included sample workout programs that you can follow. Make sure you become comfortable with the *Support & Stabilization* programs before switching over to the *Advanced Reinforcement* programs.

Shoulders

The shoulder is a complex joint with an extremely wide range of movement. It allows us to do many different kinds of movements, such as throwing a ball, reaching behind our backs, and working with objects both below and above our heads. Since it is so useful, we tend to use it a lot, and take its function for granted.

Unfortunately, its extensive mobility is also a great weakness. To allow for such a wide range of movement, the ball-and-socket joint is shallow, making it inherently less stable. Furthermore, the ligaments that hold the shoulder joint together are looser than in the hip joint, which is another ball-and-socket joint. This means that the surrounding muscles need to provide more support in order to protect the joint from the stresses imposed on it. This is why people have problems like rotator cuff strains or tears, shoulder instabilities, dislocations, and so on. If any of the shoulder muscles are weak or not properly engaged when the shoulder is being used, the joint is at increased risk for injury.

To build fundamental strength in the muscles that protect the shoulder joint, start with the Sit Press, Front Plank, Back Plank and Side Plank Progressions. As you progress to the more difficult exercises in those progressions, you will get a better feel of how to engage those muscles

Shoulder 1: OMW Support & Stabilization

Day 1	Day 2	Day 3	Day 4			
Sit Press	Front Plank	Back Plank	Side Plank	Back to Day 1		

Shoulder 2: OMW Reinforcement

Day 1	Day 2	Day 3	Day 4	Day 5	Day 6	Day 7
Sit Press	Pull-Up	Front Plank	Side Plank	Handstand	Back Plank	Front Lever
Day 8						
Back Lever	Back to Day 1					

in order to stabilize the joint under heavy loads. At that point, you can start adding Advanced Progressions such as Front Levers, Back Levers, Handstands, and Pull-Ups. These exercises will build additional strength and further teach you how to engage the necessary shoulder muscles at even higher work loads.

Elbows

The elbow is basically a hinge joint, like the hinge on a door. It mostly moves in one plane and is inherently more stable than the shoulder joint. However, it can still be injured quite easily. This usually happens when you put it under extensive stress, such as fast jerking movements, whip-like motions, excessive weight, or just plain overuse. Under these conditions, you can easily hyperextend the joint or develop tendonitis. The key is to know its natural range of motion and to build up the strength of the muscles around the joint. This way, you will recognize when to stop the joint from being strained past its limits and be strong enough to do it.

The more difficult exercises in the Front Plank, Back Plank, and Side Plank Progressions will help strengthen the elbow joint. In these exercises, you need to maintain straight arms in reverse leveraged positions. Your triceps, biceps, and forearm muscles will work intensely, balancing against each other to keep your elbows straight.

When you get stronger, you can use the Front Lever, Back Lever, Planche, and Iron Cross from the Advanced Progressions in Section V to further strengthen your elbow joint and associated muscles. Be warned that while you should never rush through any of the Progressions, it is especially critical for the Iron Cross. This set of exercises places high levels of stress on the elbow. If your muscles are not properly prepared, you can injure your elbow instead of strengthening it. Instead, take extra care to focus on good form and only progress to a more difficult exercise when you are very comfortable with the current one. Speaking from personal experience, you will benefit much more without unnecessary pain.

Elbow 1: OMW Support & Stabilization

Day 1	Day 2	Day 3				
Front Plank	Back Plank	Side Plank	Back to Day 1			

Elbow 2: OMW Reinforcement

Day 1	Day 2	Day 3	Day 4	Day 5	Day 6	Day 7
Front Plank	Back Plank	Front Lever	Side Plank	Planche	Back Lever	Iron Cross
Back to Day 1						

Hips

As a ball-and-socket joint, the hip enables you to move your legs through a wide range of motion. The ball portion is set much deeper in the socket than in the shoulder, giving the joint more stability. Despite this, hip joint issues are still fairly common, especially in this sedentary day and age.

Many muscles are involved in moving this joint, and imbalances in any one of them can lead to improper movement patterns and pain. Weakness in one muscle can overwork other muscles trying to compensate. Muscles that are not moved through their full range of motion regularly become shorter and tighter, which leads to pain and reduced function in your hip. If any of these issues manifest, it often does so silently, and grows worse until it becomes symptomatic.

All of the Basic Progressions help strengthen the muscles of the hip joint, thereby increasing stability and improving functionality. Specifically, the Sit Presses, Front, Back, and Side Planks focus just on strength. The Squats, Front Leg Raises, Back Leg Raises, Side Leg Raises, and Back Lean Leg Raises work on strength *and* control. The Front Levers, Back Levers, and Flags from the Advanced Progressions will help develop additional strength in the muscles acting on the hip joint.

Hip 1: OMW Support & Stabilization

Day 1	Day 2	Day 3	Day 4	Day 5	Day 6	Day 7
Sit Press	Squat	Front Plank	Side Leg Raise	Back Plank	Front Leg Raise	Side Plank
Day 8	**Day 9**					
Back Leg Raise	Back Lean Leg Raise	Back to Day 1				

Hip 2: OMW Reinforcement

Day 1	Day 2	Day 3	Day 4	Day 5	Day 6	Day 7
Sit Press	Squat	Front Plank	Side Leg Raise	Back Lever	Back Leg Raise	Back Plank
Day 8	**Day 9**	**Day 10**	**Day 11**	**Day 12**		
Front Leg Raise	Front Lever	Side Plank	Back Lean Leg Raise	Flag	Back to Day 1	

Knees

As one of the major shock absorbers in our body, our knees are subjected to lots of abuse. However, strong leg muscles can help absorb some of the stress and protect the knee joint. The knee is a hinge joint, but the surfaces of the knee bones are flatter than those of the elbow bones, making the joint less stable. Large ligaments, such as the Anterior Cruciate Ligament (ACL) and Posterior Cruciate Ligament (PCL), help hold the joint together and stabilize it to a certain degree. However, the knees are exposed to high loads, as well as stress from side-to-side movement. Without additional support from the surrounding muscles, these ligaments are easily overwhelmed and injured. The large quadriceps and hamstring muscles are key in providing this support. They work in opposite directions to keep the joint surfaces in place. If these muscles are weak or imbalanced, then the knee is more easily injured. Therefore, it is important to work on your leg muscles sufficiently, and in an even manner, so that they can continue to stabilize and protect your knee joint for the entire duration of the activities you plan on doing.

To strengthen your knees, start with the Squat, Front Leg Raise, Back Leg Raise, and Side Leg Raise Progressions. The Squat Progression will build fundamental strength and endurance. The leg raise exercises will work synergistically with the squat exercises to further strengthen the leg muscles and improve muscle tone. The balance aspects of these exercises will teach you how to engage your leg muscles in various body positions. When you feel strong enough, you can add the Back Lean Leg Raises, which will further strengthen your knee.

Knee 1: OMW Support & Stabilization

Day 1	Day 2	Day 3	Day 4		
Squat	Front Leg Raise	Back Leg Raise	Side Leg Raise	Back to Day 1	

Knee 2: OMW Reinforcement

Day 1	Day 2	Day 3	Day 4	Day 5	
Squat	Back Lean Leg Raise	Front Leg Raise	Back Leg Raise	Side Leg Raise	Back to Day 1

Ankles

The ankle joint allows us to move on uneven surfaces. It also assists in jumping and landing. Strong ankles are essential to effective movement and in preventing falls. If you have weak ankles, it usually means the muscles that act on that joint are weak. While you can spend a lot of time doing specific exercises to strengthen each muscle individually, it is more efficient to work on your balance. Doing so will simultaneously work on all of the muscles that protect the ankle joint. Furthermore, improving your sense of balance will enable you to gain a deeper understanding of how to adjust your body when you are about to fall. By improving the way you react, you may minimize injuries from falls, or prevent them altogether.

To work on balance, begin with the Squat, Front Leg Raise, Back Leg Raise, and Side Leg Raise Progressions. Initially, lightly hold on to a support when you do the exercises so you can focus on building strength in the appropriate muscles. As you get stronger, you can shift your focus to the small adjustments you need to make in order to maintain your balance. When you feel ready, reduce the amount of support you rely on until you are able to complete the exercises without using any supports. At that point, you can add in the Back Lean Leg Raise Progressions, which will hone your sense of balance even further.

Ankle 1: OMW Support & Stabilization

Day 1	Day 2	Day 3	Day 4			
Squat	Front Leg Raise	Back Leg Raise	Side Leg Raise	Back to Day 1		

Ankle 2: OMW Reinforcement

Day 1	Day 2	Day 3	Day 4	Day 5	
Squat	Back Lean Leg Raise	Front Leg Raise	Back Leg Raise	Side Leg Raise	Back to Day 1

Back

While you may not think of your back as a joint, it actually consists of many little joints. Each vertebra in your spine connects with its neighboring vertebra through a joint, which permits a small degree of movement. With so many vertebrae, each capable of moving a bit, the entire spine is quite flexible. Without sufficient balanced muscular support, the spinal joints are easily stressed to the point of injury.

Back pain can originate from problems in the muscles themselves, the nerves of the spinal cord, or from the bones, cartilage, and ligaments of the spine. Once you recover from an acute back injury, you need to work on strengthening the supporting muscles in a balanced manner. This means working on your core. Fortunately, every progression in the One Minute Workout works on your core. Start with the Basic Progressions in Section IV to build a solid foundation. Then, add in Advanced Progressions from Section V to further boost your strength. This will ensure that your core is strong enough to handle your body weight and activities.

Back 1: OMW Support & Stabilization

Day 1	Day 2	Day 3	Day 4	Day 5	Day 6	Day 7
Sit Press	Squat	Front Plank	Side Leg Raise	Back Plank	Front Leg Raise	Side Plank
Day 8	**Day 9**					
Back Leg Raise	Back Lean Leg Raise	Back to Day 1				

Back 2: OMW Reinforcement

Day 1	Day 2	Day 3	Day 4	Day 5	Day 6	Day 7
Sit Press	Squat	Front Plank	Hand-stand	Side Leg Raise	Planche	Back Lever
Day 8	**Day 9**	**Day 10**	**Day 11**	**Day 12**	**Day 13**	**Day 14**
Back Leg Raise	Pull-Up	Front Leg Raise	Back Plank	Front Lever	Back Lean Leg Raise	Side Plank
Day 15						
Flag	Back to Day 1					

○ 15

Improving Your Performance

This chapter is for people looking to build strength for a particular movement. Here, you will learn which progressions can be used to improve your strength in several common movements. With this guide, you will be better able to customize your workout routine for maximal benefit. Feel free to skip around to the parts that fit your needs. Remember, you can use the One Minute Workout by itself or with your current training regimen to accelerate performance improvement.

Improving Your Bench Press

The bench press focuses on chest and triceps strength, along with shoulder strength for balancing purposes. Start with the Sit Press and Front Plank Progressions. As you get stronger, you can start adding in the Planche, Handstands, and Back Levers from the Advanced Progressions.

Bench Press 1: OMW Essentials

Day 1	Day 2					
Sit Press	Front Plank	Back to Day 1				

Bench Press 2: OMW Enhanced Strength

Day 1	Day 2	Day 3	Day 4	Day 5		
Sit Press	Planche	Hand-stand	Front Plank	Back Lever	Back to Day 1	

Improving Your Shoulder Press

The shoulder press requires triceps and shoulder strength. The upper chest, trapezius, and rhomboid muscles help with stabilization. Start with the Sit Press, Front Plank, and Back Plank Progressions. These will help you develop the target muscles and the supporting muscle groups, such as the chest, upper back, and core. When you're ready, work in the Handstand Progression to mimic the shoulder press movement and the Planche to further increase shoulder strength.

Shoulder Press 1: OMW Essentials						
Day 1	Day 2	Day 3				
Sit Press	Front Plank	Back Plank	Back to Day 1			

Shoulder Press 2: OMW Enhanced Strength						
Day 1	Day 2	Day 3	Day 4	Day 5		
Sit Press	Planche	Back Plank	Handstand	Front Plank	Back to Day 1	

Improving Your Pull-Up (Vertical)

Pulling yourself up, as in a pull-up or chin-up, requires you to work in the vertical axis. This movement utilizes the biceps and upper back muscles, especially the traps, lats, and rhomboids. Although the Sit Press Progression builds pushing strength, it is an excellent one to begin with because it helps strengthen the stabilizing muscles used during pulling. Then, start adding in the Pull-Up, Front Lever and Back Lever Progressions. These will target the pulling muscles and further strengthen the stabilizing muscles. When you have nearly mastered the Pull-Up Progression, you are ready to work on the One-Arm Pull-Up Progression. You can also work in the Iron Cross Progression if you have access to rings. You will find that doing Iron Cross work will work intensely on your chest, biceps, and lats.

Vertical Pull 1: OMW Essentials

Day 1	Day 2	Day 3	Day 4			
Sit Press	Pull-Up	Front Lever	Back Lever	Back to Day 1		

Vertical Pull 2: OMW Enhanced Strength

Day 1	Day 2	Day 3	Day 4	Day 5	Day 6	
Sit Press	Pull-Up	Front Lever	Iron Cross	Back Lever	One-Arm Pull-Up	Back to Day 1

Improving Your Rowing Motion

Pulling toward yourself in a rowing motion also utilizes the biceps and upper back muscles, but at a different angle than during a pull-up. Despite the difference, the recommended progressions are identical to those for vertical pulling. Start with the Sit Press Progression to prepare your supporting muscles for strong rowing. Then, add in the Pull-Up, Front Lever and Back Lever Progressions, which will target the pulling muscles. When you are ready, you can add in the One-Arm Pull-Up Progression, as well as the Iron Cross Progression if you have access to rings.

Rowing 1: OMW Essentials

Day 1	Day 2	Day 3	Day 4			
Sit Press	Pull-Up	Front Lever	Back Lever	Back to Day 1		

Rowing 2: OMW Enhanced Strength

Day 1	Day 2	Day 3	Day 4	Day 5	Day 6	
Sit Press	Pull-Up	Front Lever	Iron Cross	Back Lever	One-Arm Pull-Up	Back to Day 1

Improving Your Bicep Curl

The curling motion focuses primarily on the biceps. The Pull-Up and One-Arm Pull-Up Progressions directly target the biceps, especially in the bent arm positions. The Front Plank and Back Lever Progressions also work on the biceps, but in a straight arm position, which produces massive strength gains. Again, if you have access to exercise rings, the Iron Cross Progression is an excellent way to train your biceps while working the rest of your upper body simultaneously.

Bicep Curl 1: OMW Essentials

Day 1	Day 2	Day 3				
Pull-Up	Front Plank	Back Lever	Back to Day 1			

Bicep Curl 2: OMW Enhanced Strength

Day 1	Day 2	Day 3	Day 4	Day 5		
Pull-Up	Front Plank	Back Lever	One-Arm Pull-Up	Iron Cross	Back to Day 1	

Improving Your Hanging

Hanging from a support, such as a bar or ledge, requires good upper back and grip strength. Doing the Pull-Up and One-Arm Pull-Up Progressions will help tremendously in your ability to hang. However,

Hanging 1: OMW Essentials

Day 1	Day 2	Day 3				
Pull-Up	Front Lever	Back Lever	Back to Day 1			

Hanging 2: OMW Enhanced Strength

Day 1	Day 2	Day 3	Day 4			
Pull-Up	Front Lever	One-Arm Pull-Up	Back Lever	Back to Day 1		

you should also work on the Front and Back Lever Progressions, since these will improve your ability to shift your body into different positions while hanging.

Improving Your Abdominal Flexion (Crunch Movement)

Doing an abdominal crunch or sit-up works on the abdominal muscles, and to a lesser extent, the oblique muscles. All of the progressions in this book will work on the abs, but if you want to focus on them intensely, Sit Presses, Front Planks, and Back Lean Leg Raises are good places to start. As you become stronger, work in the Front Lever and Planche Progressions. These two will give your abs an intense workout. You can also throw in the Flag and Side Plank Progressions to work on the obliques and abdominals at the same time.

Ab Flexion 1: OMW Essentials

Day 1	Day 2	Day 3				
Sit Press	Front Plank	Back Lean Leg Raise	Back to Day 1			

Ab Flexion 2: OMW Enhanced Strength

Day 1	Day 2	Day 3	Day 4	Day 5	Day 6	Day 7
Sit Press	Planche	Back Lean Leg Raise	Front Plank	Flag	Front Lever	Side Plank
Back to Day 1						

Improving Your Lifting

Lifting things, such as heavy boxes or furniture, requires strong legs as well as a strong core and upper body. Many people lift objects with incorrect form and end up hurting their backs. The best thing that you can do to prevent these kinds of injuries is to use proper lifting form and only lift as much as you can comfortably handle. Proper lifting form generally involves squatting down, getting a good grip, and lifting with your legs while keeping your back straight and upright. If the object is too heavy, ask other people to help you lift it. While you may feel that getting help from others is inconvenient, just think about how inconvenient the rest of your life could be if you end up hurting your back permanently. As a doctor, I have seen countless patients who have hurt their backs unnecessarily. There is absolutely no shame in asking for help when it comes to protecting your health.

As for recommended progressions, all of the progressions in this book work on core strength. Make sure you work through the Basic Progressions from Section IV. The Sit Press, Front Plank, Back Plank, and Side Plank Progressions will target the upper body, while the other progressions target the lower body. The Back Lean Leg Raises will provide additional focus on the core.

Lifting 1: OMW Essentials

Day 1	Day 2	Day 3	Day 4	Day 5	Day 6	Day 7
Sit Press	Squat	Front Plank	Side Leg Raise	Back Plank	Front Leg Raise	Side Plank
Day 8	**Day 9**					
Back Leg Raise	Back Lean Leg Raise	Back to Day 1				

Lifting 2: OMW Enhanced Strength

Day 1	Day 2	Day 3	Day 4	Day 5	Day 6	Day 7
Sit Press	Squat	Front Plank	Hand-stand	Side Leg Raise	Planche	Back Lever
Day 8	**Day 9**	**Day 10**	**Day 11**	**Day 12**	**Day 13**	**Day 14**
Back Leg Raise	Pull-Up	Front Leg Raise	Back Plank	Front Lever	Iron Cross	Back Lean Leg Raise
Day 15	**Day 16**	**Day 17**				
Side Plank	Flag	One-Arm Pull-Up	Back to Day 1			

Improving Your Squatting

Squatting requires strength in all of your lower body muscles, but focuses a lot on the quads, hamstrings and glutes. Not surprisingly, the Squat Progression is perfect for working on squatting. The Front Leg Raise, Back Leg Raise, and Side Leg Raise Progressions will also help with the squatting movement by improving your balance and strengthening the supporting muscle groups.

Squatting: OMW Essentials

Day 1	Day 2	Day 3	Day 4			
Squat	Front Leg Raise	Back Leg Raise	Side Leg Raise	Back to Day 1		

Improving Your Balance (Strengthening Your Ankle)

Balancing requires good body awareness and enough strength in the lower body to properly compensate for any changes. Use the Squat Progression to build basic leg strength and the Front Leg Raise, Back Leg Raise, and Side Leg Raise Progressions to improve your ankle strength, balance, and reflexes. As you become more proficient, you can add in the Back Lean Leg Raises. For all of these Progressions, start off using a support if needed and then wean yourself from it as soon as you are comfortable. Doing so will give you the maximum benefit in the least amount of time.

Balance (Ankle): OMW Essentials

Day 1	Day 2	Day 3	Day 4	Day 5		
Squat	Front Leg Raise	Back Leg Raise	Side Leg Raise	Back Lean Leg Raise	Back to Day 1	

Improving Your Jumping

Jumping is a complex movement that requires coordination of the upper body and explosive strength from the lower body. Work on the Squat Progression for raw lower body strength. You can also add in the

Front Leg Raise, Back Leg Raise, and Side Leg Raise Progressions to further improve lower body strength. They will also help improve your balance and reflexes.

Jumping: OMW Essentials

Day 1	Day 2	Day 3	Day 4			
Squat	Front Leg Raise	Back Leg Raise	Side Leg Raise	Back to Day 1		

Improving Your Kicking

Kicking is a complex movement that can easily throw you off balance. Good kicking technique requires coordination of the upper body and strength in the lower body. The Front Leg Raise, Back Leg Raise, Side Leg Raise, and Back Lean Leg Raise Progressions will develop the strength and balance needed for these movements. Work on the Squat Progression to further enhance your kicking power.

Also, consider adding some core and upper body work for specific types of kicks. I suggest working on Sit Presses, Front Planks, and Front Levers for front kicks. For roundhouse kicks, add Side Planks and Flags to the suggestions for front kicks. These will help increase

Kicking: OMW Essentials

Day 1	Day 2	Day 3	Day 4	Day 5		
Squat	Front Leg Raise	Back Leg Raise	Side Leg Raise	Back Lean Leg Raise	Back to Day 1	

Front Kick: OMW Enhanced Strength

Day 1	Day 2	Day 3	Day 4	Day 5	Day 6	Day 7
Squat	Sit Press	Front Leg Raise	Front Plank	Back Leg Raise	Front Lever	Side Leg Raise
Day 8						
Back Lean Leg Raise	Back to Day 1					

rotational power. For back kicks, work on the Back Plank and Back Lever. The Side Plank and Flag Progressions will enhance side kicks as well as spinning-type kicks.

Roundhouse Kick: OMW Enhanced Strength

Day 1	Day 2	Day 3	Day 4	Day 5	Day 6	Day 7
Squat	Sit Press	Front Leg Raise	Front Plank	Side Leg Raise	Front Lever	Back Leg Raise

Day 8	Day 9	Day 10				
Side Plank	Back Lean Leg Raise	Flag	Back to Day 1			

Back Kick: OMW Enhanced Strength

Day 1	Day 2	Day 3	Day 4	Day 5	Day 6	Day 7
Squat	Back Plank	Front Leg Raise	Back Lever	Back Leg Raise	Side Leg Raise	Back Lean Leg Raise
Back to Day 1						

Spinning Kicks: OMW Enhanced Strength

Day 1	Day 2	Day 3	Day 4	Day 5	Day 6	Day 7
Squat	Side Plank	Back Leg Raise	Flag	Front Leg Raise	Side Leg Raise	Back Lean Leg Raise
Back to Day 1						

Side Kick: OMW Enhanced Strength

Day 1	Day 2	Day 3	Day 4	Day 5	Day 6	Day 7
Squat	Side Plank	Back Leg Raise	Flag	Front Leg Raise	Side Leg Raise	Back Lean Leg Raise
Back to Day 1						

Improving Your Punching

Effective punching requires coordination of the entire body and power in both the extension and retraction phases. You will need to do both pushing and pulling exercises. Real power in a punch doesn't come just from the arms, but starts from your legs and transfers through your core and upper body before reaching your fists. All of the Progressions in this book will help improve these areas. The Sit Press, Front Plank, Back Plank, and Pull-Up Progressions are good places to start for the upper body. The Squat, Front Leg Raise, and Back Leg Raise Progressions are good starting points for the lower body. Add in the Side Planks and Flags to increase rotational power.

Punching: OMW Essentials						
Day 1	Day 2	Day 3	Day 4	Day 5	Day 6	Day 7
Sit Press	Squat	Front Plank	Hand-stand	Side Leg Raise	Planche	Back Lever
Day 8	Day 9	Day 10	Day 11	Day 12	Day 13	Day 14
Back Leg Raise	Pull-Up	Front Leg Raise	Back Plank	Front Lever	Iron Cross	Back Lean Leg Raise
Day 15	Day 16	Day 17				
Side Plank	Flag	One-Arm Pull-Up	Back to Day 1			

Section IV

Basic Progressions
&
Exercises

16

Getting Started

All right! Are you ready to start your first One Minute Workout? From here on, you will find detailed information about each progression and the exercises it encompasses. There is no need to read these chapters straight through. The information is laid out so these pages can be used as a training guide. Details are repeated where relevant so you can jump straight to the exercise you want and get started quickly. Make things even easier by using sticky notes to bookmark the pages with the exercises that you are working on. You can also write down your progress for each exercise on these sticky notes. This way, when you look back over your workout history, you can see how much you have improved. Reviewing your progress is a great way to keep yourself motivated.

Remember that in the One Minute Workout, a **Progression** is a set of related **Exercises** organized by difficulty. Each progression targets a different set of muscles in a unique way. The progressions are split into two groups, the Basic Progressions and the Advanced Progressions. The Basic Progressions will help you build a solid, well-rounded foundation of strength. They are recommended for everyone. The Advanced Progressions will build tremendous strength and are intended for those looking for a challenge and to maximize their physical performance.

Summary of the Workout Routine

In case you skipped the "How It Works" chapter, let's review the workout routine. Each day, you only need to do a single exercise from just one of the progressions, for a total of one minute. Keep in mind that it is okay to break up the minute into a few sessions. This is actually expected when you are working on an exercise of the appropriate difficulty. Just hold the exercise position for as long as you can during each exercise session. As you get stronger, you'll be able to hold the position longer and longer.

Eventually, you will grow strong enough to finish the entire minute in a single session. This means you have mastered that exercise. The next time you work on the same progression, you are ready to advance to a more difficult exercise.

Don't forget to pick a different progression from the one you did the day before. This way, you will cycle through the progressions and train your muscles in a different way each day. Over time, you will build a good foundation of all-around strength.

Tracking Your Workout and Progress

When you find the exercise in a progression that fits your current strength level, bookmark it with a sticky note or a slip of paper so you can find that exercise quickly in the future. You can also jot down your workout session durations on the bookmark. When you master the exercise, take the old bookmark out and put a new one on the next exercise in the progression. This is a simple way to keep track of where you are in each progression so you don't need to rely on your memory.

Alternatively, you can use the One Minute Workout Tracker worksheets found in the Appendix. Each day, write the exercise name in a new row and jot down each workout session in the appropriate box on the worksheet. If you prefer to track your workout electronically and get workout reminders sent to you, visit the One Minute Workout website at www.OneMinWorkout.com. There, you will find the tools that I personally use for my workouts.

Choosing Your Progressions

Before you start your first workout, you should decide which progressions you want to put in your rotation. Picking your progressions enables you to customize your workout to target desired effects, such as strengthening a weak joint, or improving a particular movement. For suggestions on specific goals, refer to "Chapter 14: Fixing Your Body" and "Chapter 15: Improving Your Performance." Otherwise, if you are looking for a balanced workout, you can try the suggestions below. Once you have picked out your progressions, write them down in a list. This way, you can just go down the list, doing one progression each day.

If you are new to working out, I recommend starting with the following essential Basic Progressions:

1. Sit Presses
2. Squats
3. Front Planks
4. Front Leg Raises
5. Back Planks

You can program your workouts as shown below or make up your own program.

OMW Essential Basics						
Monday	**Tuesday**	**Wednesday**	**Thursday**	**Friday**	**Saturday**	**Sunday**
Sit Press	Squat	Front Plank	Front Leg Raise	Back Plank	Rest	Rest

These will help you build a solid foundation of strength and balance that will help you in whatever activities you do in the future. If you want to develop a lot of all-around strength, try rotating through all of the Basic Progressions:

1. Sit Presses
2. Squats
3. Front Plank
4. Front Leg Raises
5. Back Plank
6. Back Leg Raises
7. Side Plank
8. Side Leg Raises
9. Back Lean Leg Raises

The following is a sample workout program that includes all of the Basic Progressions. Note that this example covers two full cycles.

Basic
Progressions

OMW All Basics

Monday	Tuesday	Wednesday	Thursday	Friday	Saturday	Sunday
Sit Press	Squat	Front Plank	Side Leg Raise	Back Plank	Front Leg Raise	Rest

Monday	Tuesday	Wednesday	Thursday	Friday	Saturday	Sunday
Side Plank	Back Leg Raise	Back Lean Leg Raise	Sit Press	Squat	Front Plank	Rest

Monday	Tuesday	Wednesday	Thursday	Friday	Saturday	Sunday
Side Leg Raise	Back Plank	Front Leg Raise	Side Plank	Back Leg Raise	Back Lean Leg Raise	Rest

Working on all of the Basic Progressions will ensure a strong solid core and a high level of strength in all of your major muscle groups. These exercises will not require any specialized equipment.

If you want to develop exceptional strength, then you should rotate through all of the Basic Progressions as well as the Advanced Progressions found in Section V. Most of the Advanced Progressions will require at least a support that you can hang from, such as a pull-up bar. See the "Introduction to the Advanced Progressions" chapter for more details.

If you have many progressions in your rotation, you will need to consider how long it takes for you to rotate back to the first one. If you don't work out a muscle group for a while, you will start to lose some of the progress you have made. Exactly how long it takes for this to happen varies from person to person, although 14 days is about average. Many of the exercises in the progressions work on overlapping muscle groups so you may not lose progress that fast. However, if you are looking to develop peak functional strength, you should aim to repeat a specific progression no more than 14 days later. If you have too many progressions in your rotation, try taking some of the easier ones out. Alternatively, if you have time, you can do more than one progression a day. This way, you can rotate through all of them in less than 14 days.

Basic Progressions

Picking Your First Exercise in a Progression

When you work on a progression for the first time, you will need to find the exercise that is appropriate for your current strength level. You don't necessarily need to start at the first level exercise in each progression. A good rule of thumb is to pick an exercise that you can hold for at least five seconds, but not more than one minute continuously. If you can do the whole minute continuously, then choose the next exercise in the progression.

If you are not in shape, pick one near the beginning of the progression. If you are in average shape, try something in the middle. If you are already really strong, you can try one of the later exercises. You can also use the recommendations shown on the exercise map at the beginning of each progression chapter. Whichever one you pick, check to see how the exercise feels and move up or down in difficulty as appropriate.

Exercise Difficulty Ratings

I have assigned a difficulty rating to each exercise in this book. These are estimates of how difficult one exercise is relative to the others, based on my experience. Because each person's body is unique, your experience may be different. You may also notice that two sequential exercises in a progression have been assigned the same difficulty rating. This does not mean that they are the same difficulty, just that they are close enough to be in the same tier. Remember that exercises further along in a progression are always harder than earlier ones.

Basic Progressions

Do I Need to Work Through Every Exercise in a Progression?

The short answer is no. Just progress through the exercises in a progression until you have reached the results you desire. Then, maintain what you have achieved by sticking with that exercise. Keep in mind that significant functional benefit can be gained from even the mid-level exercises.

The more difficult the exercise, the more strength and muscle you will build. If you are looking to gain a lot of strength and muscle, then you will want to progress as far as you can. On the other hand, if you are looking to maintain what you have now, you can stay with a suitably difficult exercise in the progression. You can always change your mind later and move on to a more difficult exercise.

What Do These Exercises Feel Like?

The answer to this question will vary, because each person has a different strength profile. For example, some people have strong cores and weak arms, while others have strong legs and weaker upper bodies. That being said, you can expect these exercises to work the target muscles quite intensely, especially when you are pushing yourself to expand your limits. You may feel a burning sensation in your muscles as you perform the exercises, especially in the bigger muscles, such as the quads. The more muscles you engage, the more effort it will take. You may even feel your body temperature rise after an exercise session. Don't worry. This is normal and is the result of the intense contractions of a large number of muscles at the same time.

It is also normal to feel a little shaky or wobbly during the exercise, especially as you get tired. This is a sign that you have worked your muscles nearly to their limits. The shakiness will go away as you get stronger. The same thing goes for mild cramping while exercising, especially in the quads and triceps. These cramps should go away shortly after you stop the exercise. They will also go away as you get stronger. However, if the cramps don't go away quickly, then it may be a sign that you have overworked some muscles. Try stretching and massaging the affected muscles lightly. If they do not feel better in a few days, consult your physician.

On the other hand, feeling joint pain is NOT normal. If you feel pain in your joints, stop immediately. Chances are, your muscles are not ready to support your joints in that exercise. Switch to an easier exercise and work on it more until you build up the muscles that stabilize the joint. If the pain is in the wrists, you can also try changing the position of your hands to see if the pain goes away.

Remember to Breathe!

Just because these exercises are static holds doesn't mean you should hold your breath while doing them. Your muscles need all the blood flow they can get in order to perform optimally, especially when an exercise lasts longer than the anaerobic phase. Holding your breath while exerting temporarily reduces the amount of blood pumped by your heart, thereby decreasing the blood flow to your muscles. To prevent this and to improve performance, make sure you keep breathing while exercising.

Right before doing an exercise, take a few deep breaths to prime your body with oxygen and to get rid of some extra carbon dioxide. Then, breathe out as you contract your muscles and start the exercise. Focus on breathing regularly as you continue doing the exercise. If the exercise is so intense that you can't breathe regularly, take shallow breaths instead.

Can I Do More Than One Minute a Day?

If you are the go-getter type and want to go above and beyond the one minute for an exercise, you are by all means welcome to. This is called **supercharging** an exercise and can help build strength even faster. Just don't go crazy with it and do the exercise for too long, since there are diminishing returns after a certain amount of time. I recommend limiting supercharging to a maximum of one additional minute. Similarly, if you want to do more than one exercise from different Progressions in a single day, that is fine too. Be sure to listen to your body and make sure you give it enough time to recover from your workouts so that you don't end up overtraining and get hurt.

How Your Height and Weight Affect the Exercises

Since these exercises are bodyweight exercises, your weight will obviously affect difficulty. However, these exercises also depend on the principles of leverage. Therefore, your height and other body dimensions also affect difficulty. In general, the taller you are, the longer your arms and legs are. This means the amount of leverage working against your muscles will be greater than for someone with shorter body dimensions. This is one of the reasons that elite gymnasts tend to be smaller. Since they tend to perform leveraged bodyweight-based techniques, a smaller body size reduces the leverage working against their muscles.

If you want to compete with your friends to see who can go fastest through these progressions, be sure to keep the above points in mind. Do not become discouraged if any of your physically smaller friends seem to be progressing faster. The increased weight and leverage working against your longer limbs means that you actually develop greater absolute strength with the same exercises.

Optional Specialized Equipment

The Basic Progressions in the One Minute Workout were designed not to require any specialized equipment. Most of these exercises simply require some floor space or a chair. However, if you want to use some optional equipment as aids, to provide variety, or even to increase the difficulty of the exercises, feel free to be creative and make use of whatever is around you, as long as it is stable and safe. For example, you can use a set of heavy books or a pair of stationary chairs instead of push-up handles or paralletes.

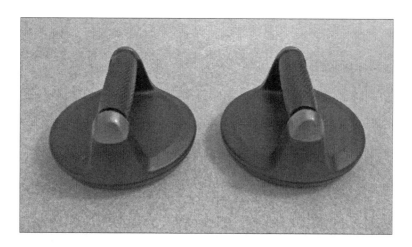

Push-Up Handles

These portable units are usually made of plastic or metal and come in a variety of sizes and designs. Find a set that feels comfortable when you use it. Also, check to make sure that it has a stable base. You don't want it to fall over in the middle of an exercise. If you want to increase the difficulty of your exercises, you can also opt for push-up handles that rotate, such as the ones shown. The extra bit of instability will engage more of your muscles and give them a better workout.

Paralletes

Paralletes are miniature versions of the parallel bars you see in gymnastics. They are similar to push-up handles, but are generally taller and have bigger handles. I've seen them range from just a few inches tall to over 18 inches tall. The ones I use at home (pictured below) are about 11 inches tall and 17 inches long. The extra height gives you more clearance from the ground to work with. For example, you can use them for Sit Presses to make it easier to keep your feet off the ground. You can also use them to raise your feet off the ground to make exercises like the Front and Back Planks harder.

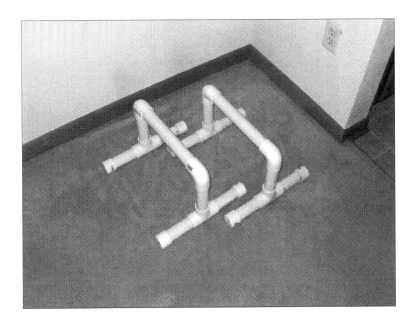

They come in a variety of materials, including wood, plastic, and metal. You can buy them online or at some sports equipment stores but if you are handy, you can easily make them in any size you want. All you need is some PVC piping, which you can get at the hardware store. Construction instructions are available online. I prefer using 1.25 inch diameter PVC pipes for paralletes because they feel more comfortable in my hands. However, some people may prefer 1.5 inch diameter PVC pipes.

17

Sit Presses

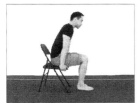
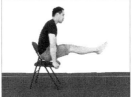
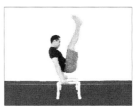

Beginner   Mid-Level   Advanced

The Sit Press Progression consists of functional exercises similar to actions we take frequently, such as getting up out of a chair, getting up off the ground, and sitting up. This is an excellent progression to start with whether you are in or out of shape. The exercises are simple and build the necessary foundation of strength for more advanced progressions. If you only do one progression from the One Minute Workout system, this is the one to do.

This progression starts in positions that mimic the movement of getting up from a chair. These exercises will strengthen the pushing muscle groups in your upper body. At this stage, you can use your legs to assist with balance, and to provide some support. As you advance through the exercises, you'll be supporting your entire body weight on just your hands. This develops your core strength (abs and back) and helps with balance and stabilization. The most difficult exercises focus intensely on the triceps, shoulders, and abs and will further develop your ability to balance yourself on your hands. By the end of this progression, you will have sculpted triceps, abs, chest and shoulder muscles.

Equipment Needed

Chair or other sitting surface

Many of the Sit Press exercises can be conveniently performed in a chair. However, you can use other kinds of supports, such as the floor, the lower steps on a set of stairs, parallettes, push-up handles, dumbbells, or rings. The difficulty will change depending on the support you use. Generally, the floor and rings will make the exercises harder since you have less clearance on the floor and less stability on the rings.

General Notes

When you do these exercises, be sure to keep your shoulders pressed down away from your ears so that you work on your shoulder girdle muscles. Doing so stabilizes your shoulder joints, enabling you to better engage your pushing muscles. This seemingly small detail will make a world of difference, especially when you get to the advanced exercises.

If you have weak rotator cuff muscles, these exercises will help strengthen them without causing too much strain. They will also help improve the stability of your shoulder joints.

Exercise Map

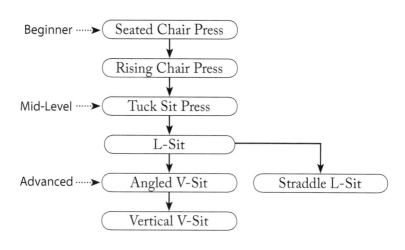

Seated Chair Press

Difficulty: ★☆☆☆☆

Directions

While sitting on a chair, place your hands by your thighs. Keeping your elbows straight, press down on the chair with your hands until you feel tension in your arms. Your butt may stay in contact with the chair, but you should feel some to most of your weight being supported by your arms and hands.

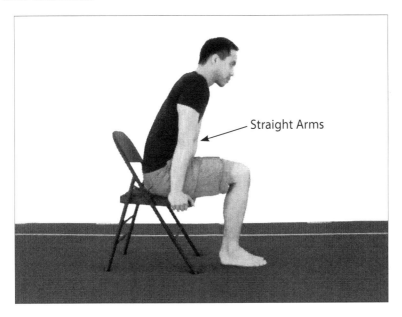

— Straight Arms

Basic Progressions

Comments

This exercise prepares you for more advanced exercises by working on your pushing muscles including the triceps, chest, upper back, and shoulder girdle muscles. You'll develop strength in those muscles without needing to support your entire body weight or worry about balance issues.

Tips

» Too easy? Instead of placing your hands by your thighs, try moving them back toward your butt. This will engage your upper back muscles more and make this exercise more difficult.

Seated Chair Press

Muscles Worked

Front: Pectorals, Front Deltoids

Back: Rotator Cuff, Triceps, Trapezius, Lats, Rhomboids

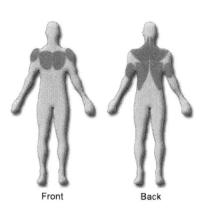

Front   Back

Rising Chair Press

Difficulty: ★☆☆☆☆

Directions

While sitting on a chair, place your hands by your thighs. Keeping your elbows straight, press down on the chair with your hands until you feel tension in your arms. Squeeze your abs and raise your butt off the chair while keeping your feet lightly on the ground. You should be supporting most of your weight on your hands. Your feet will provide the rest of the support and assist with your balance, but they should not actively push down on the floor.

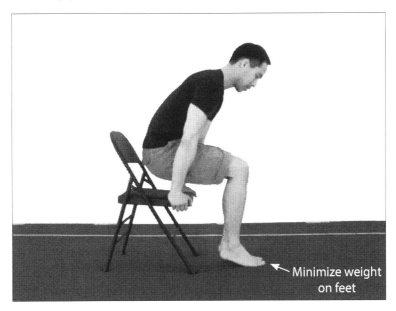

← Minimize weight on feet

Comments

This exercise increases the load on your pushing muscles and also works on your abs. If you can do this exercise fairly easily, then you should be able to get out of a chair without any problems.

Tips

» If you have trouble with this exercise at first, you can shift more of your weight to your feet. However, make sure that you squeeze your abs and push down with your hands so that your butt is off the chair. As you get stronger, start reducing the amount of support you're getting from your feet until eventually, your toes barely touch the ground.

» Too easy? Instead of placing your hands by your thighs, move them back toward your butt. This will engage your upper back muscles more and make this exercise a bit more difficult.

Muscles Worked

Front: Pectorals, Front Deltoids, Abdominals

Back: Rotator Cuff, Triceps, Trapezius, Lats, Rhomboids

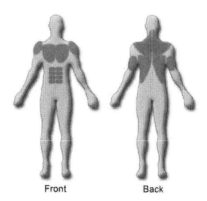

Front   Back

Tuck Sit Press

Difficulty: ★★☆☆☆

Directions

While sitting, place your hands by your thighs. Keeping your elbows straight, press down on the chair with your hands until you feel tension in your arms. Raise your butt off the chair and lift your feet off the floor by squeezing your abs and hip flexors. All of your weight should now be balanced on your hands.

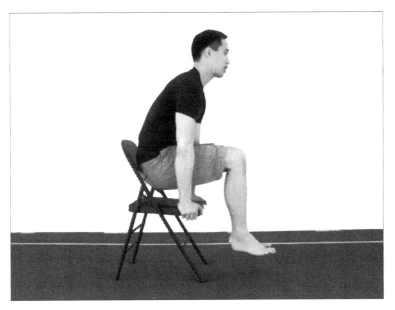

Comments

This exercise further increases the load on your pushing muscles. Since your feet and butt no longer provide support, your core muscles will need to work harder to keep your body in the proper position. It's normal to feel some cramping in your abs at first as it means they're getting a great workout. This feeling should go away as you get stronger.

Tips

  » Can't get off the chair? At this difficulty level and up, it is very important to keep your shoulders pressed down. Aside from training the proper muscles, this will increase the height you can lift your body off of the support surface. This additional clearance will be of great help when you get tired during an exercise and your body starts sagging lower.

» Too easy? Instead of placing your hands by your thighs, move them back toward your butt. Doing so will require you to push your lower body forward a bit and lean back with the upper body. This will increase the load on your triceps. You will also need to push down harder to raise your butt off of the supporting surface.

Muscles Worked

Front: Pectorals, Front Deltoids, Abdominals, Obliques, Serratus, Hip Flexors

Back: Rear Deltoids, Rotator Cuff, Triceps, Trapezius, Lats, Rhomboids, Lower Back

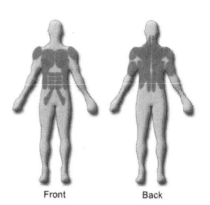

Front   Back

L-Sit

Difficulty: ★★★☆☆

Directions

While sitting, place your hands by your thighs. Keeping your elbows straight, press down on the chair with your hands until you feel tension in your arms. Raise your butt off the chair and contract your abs, hip flexors, and quads to lift your legs straight up in front of you. All of your weight should now be balanced on your hands and your legs should be parallel to the ground.

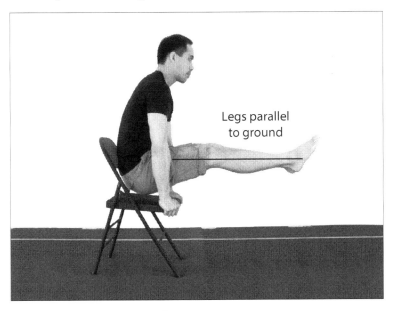

Legs parallel to ground

Basic Progressions

Comments

At this level, your abs, hip flexors and quads will all be working really hard to keep your legs horizontal. It is normal to feel some cramping in the quads when doing this exercise the first few times as it means they're getting a great workout. This feeling should go away as your muscles grow stronger.

Tips

» Too easy? Instead of placing your hands by your thighs, move them back toward your butt. This increases the difficulty in the same way as with the previous exercises, but to a greater degree. This means you will obtain better results faster.

» Still too easy? Try doing it on the floor. Being closer to the ground means you'll have to work extra hard to make sure your legs don't accidently touch the ground.

Muscles Worked

Front: Pectorals, Front Deltoids, Abdominals, Obliques, Serratus, Hip Flexors, Hip Adductors, Quads

Back: Rear Deltoids, Rotator Cuff, Triceps, Trapezius, Lats, Rhomboids, Lower Back

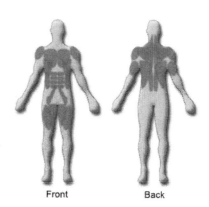

Front   Back

Straddle L-Sit

Difficulty: ★★★⯪☆

Directions

While sitting, place your hands by your thighs. Keeping your elbows straight, press down on the chair with your hands until you feel tension in your arms. Raise your butt off the chair and squeeze your abs, hip flexors, and quads to lift your legs up in front of you. Spread your legs apart into a straddle position. All of your weight should now be balanced on your hands and your legs should be parallel to the ground.

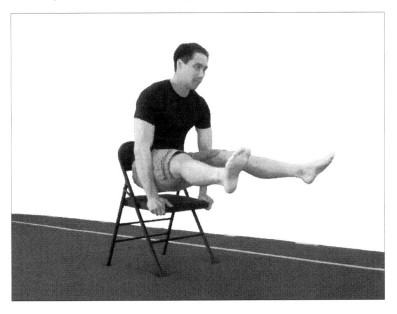

Comments

An alternate way to do this exercise is to straddle your legs with your arms *between* your legs. This will require some more leg flexibility and additional hip flexor and quad strength. Avoid resting your legs against your arms because that reduces the difficulty of this exercise. You may find that you will need to raise your lower body higher and push your butt further back to do this variation. If your chair has a back rest, this movement may be limited by the depth of the chair seat.

Tips

» If you are in the straddle position with your hands outside your legs, your arms may limit how far you can spread your legs. You can push your body forward to provide more freedom in the width of the straddle. Keep in mind that doing so will increase the difficulty of this exercise.

Variations

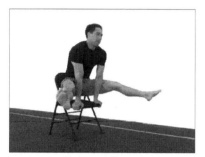

Outside Straddle on Chair

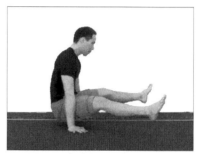

Inside Straddle on Floor

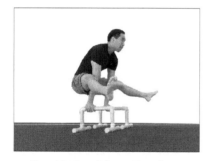

Outside Straddle on Paralletes

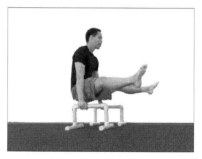

Inside Straddle on Paralletes

Muscles Worked

Front: Pectorals, Front Deltoids, Abdominals, Obliques, Serratus, Hip Flexors, Hip Adductors, Quads

Back: Rear Deltoids, Rotator Cuff, Triceps, Trapezius, Lats, Rhomboids, Lower Back, Hip Abductors

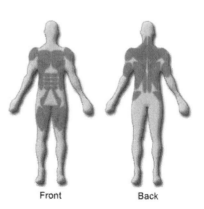

Front   Back

Basic Progressions

Angled V-Sit

Difficulty: ★★★★☆

Directions

While sitting, place your hands by your butt. Keeping your elbows straight, press down on the surface with your hands. Raise your butt off the chair and squeeze your abs, hip flexors and quads to lift your legs straight up in front of you at about a 45-degree angle to the ground. You may need to push your hips forward to help raise your feet higher.

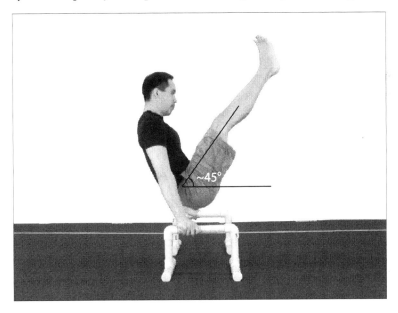

Comments

At this level, your triceps and abs will be working extremely hard due to the forward positioning of the hips.

Tips

»   Having trouble with balance? Try leaning back a little to help maintain your balance.

»   Can't get your legs high enough? Besides strength, flexibility also plays an important role here. The more flexible you are in your hamstrings and lower back, the easier it will be for your abs and hip flexors to bring your legs up. If flexibility is your problem, try stretching lightly before doing this exercise.

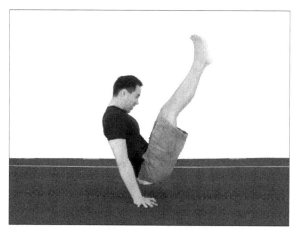

Angled V-Sit on Floor

Muscles Worked

Front: Pectorals, Front Deltoids, Abdominals, Obliques, Serratus, Hip Flexors, Hip Adductors, Quads

Back: Rear Deltoids, Rotator Cuff, Triceps, Trapezius, Lats, Rhomboids, Lower Back, Hip Abductors

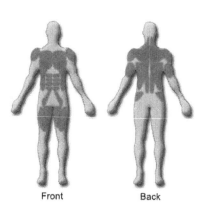

Front   Back

Vertical V-Sit

Difficulty: ★★★★★

Directions

While sitting, place your hands by your butt. Keeping your elbows straight, press down on the surface with your hands. Raise your butt off the chair and squeeze your abs, hip flexors, and quads strongly to lift your legs straight up in front of you, perpendicular to the ground. You may need to push your hips forward to help raise your feet higher.

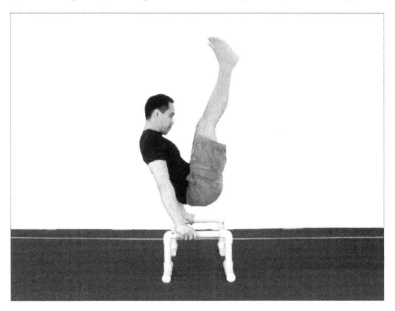

Basic Progressions

Comments

This exercise is similar to the previous one but requires an even more intense contraction of the involved muscles.

Tips

» Having trouble with balance? Try leaning back a little to help maintain your balance.

» Can't get your legs high enough? Besides strength, flexibility also plays an important role here. The more flexible you are in your hamstrings and lower back, the easier it will be for your abs and hip flexors to bring your legs up. If flexibility is your problem, try stretching lightly before doing this exercise.

Muscles Worked

Front: Pectorals, Front Deltoids, Abdominals, Obliques, Serratus, Hip Flexors, Hip Adductors, Quads

Back: Rear Deltoids, Rotator Cuff, Triceps, Trapezius, Lats, Rhomboids, Lower Back, Hip Abductors

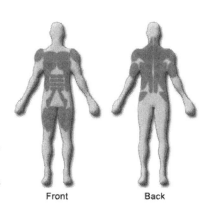

Front   Back

18

Front Planks

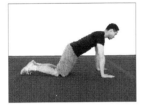 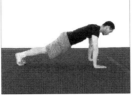 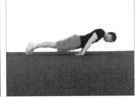

Beginner   Mid-Level   Advanced

The Front Plank Progression is an excellent way to build your core strength, especially if you are out of shape. It also builds functional strength in your upper body's pushing muscle groups. Finally, it will help firm up problem areas such as the triceps, abs, and buttocks. Balance does not play much of a role until the most advanced exercises in this progression.

A front plank looks like the upper position of the classic push-up exercise. It is important to keep your abs contracted so that your body is fully straight, or just slightly hollowed out. If you hollow your body too much so that your butt is sticking up, the effectiveness of these exercises is greatly reduced. On the other hand, if you let your abs loosen up, your back muscles will need to take on the majority of the effort. This also reduces the effectiveness of these exercises and can lead to injury. In fact, this is what happens to many people who lack core strength. Whether standing or sitting, weak abdominal muscle tone leads to poor posture, which can overwork the back muscles. Over time, they become tight and pain develops. So if you have back pain, it is time for you to take a look at your core strength and perhaps improve it.

Equipment Needed

Floor space

These exercises are usually performed on the floor, but you can also use bar-type handles or even low hanging rings. If you have wrist problems, it may be difficult for you to support your weight with your hands on the floor. In this case, you can try using push-up handles. These handles will allow you to keep your wrists in a neutral position. Working with rings will make the exercises more difficult, but your stabilizing muscles will develop faster. This is beneficial to your shoulder joints since they will become stronger and more resistant to injury.

General Notes

If you have rotator cuff issues, the front plank exercises are a good way to strengthen the muscles around the shoulder. Since these exercises are static, you will be better able to focus on muscle recruitment and body position. You will also run a lower chance of irritating old or nagging injuries compared to dynamic exercises. In addition, you will develop a better feel for how the muscles in your body work. This is critical to improving athletic ability and reducing risk of injury in the future.

Exercise Map

Beginner ┈┈▶ Front Bent Plank
↓
Mid-Level & Advanced ┈┈▶ Front Knee Plank
↓
Front Plank

Front Plank: Arms Back Lv1	Front Plank: Arms Forward Lv1	Front Plank: Arms Side Lv1
Front Plank: Arms Back Lv2	Front Plank: Arms Forward Lv2	Front Plank: Arms Side Lv2
Front Plank: Arms Back Lv3	Front Plank: Arms Forward Lv3	Front Plank: Arms Side Lv3

Basic Progressions

Front Bent Plank

Difficulty: ★☆☆☆☆

Directions

Place your hands shoulder-width apart on the ground in front of you. Rest your weight on your hands and knees. Move your knees back so that the angle between your thighs and your trunk is about 135 degrees. Make sure to keep your shoulders directly over your hands.

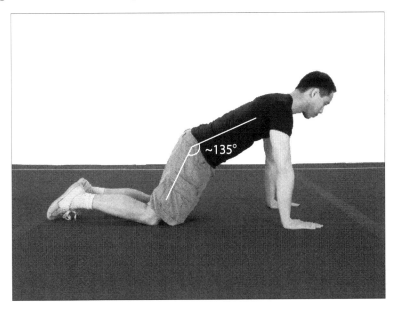

Comments

While this position is similar to resting on your hands and knees, moving your knees back a bit will require you to start contracting your abs in order to maintain the position. At the same time, it will also increase the amount of weight on your hands. If you are just beginning to work out or lacking in strength, this is an excellent exercise to start with. Stick with it for a while and before you know it, you will be able to move on to the next exercise.

Front Bent Plank

Muscles Worked

Front: Pectorals, Front Deltoids, Abdominals, Obliques, Serratus

Back: Rotator Cuff, Triceps, Trapezius, Lats, Rhomboids, Lower Back, Gluteus Maximus

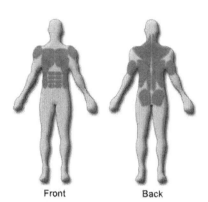

Front   Back

Front Knee Plank

Difficulty: ★☆☆☆☆

Directions

Place your hands shoulder-width apart on the ground in front of you. Rest your weight on your hands and knees. Move your knees back so that your thighs and upper body are in a straight line. Your knees should still be bent. Make sure to keep your shoulders directly over your hands.

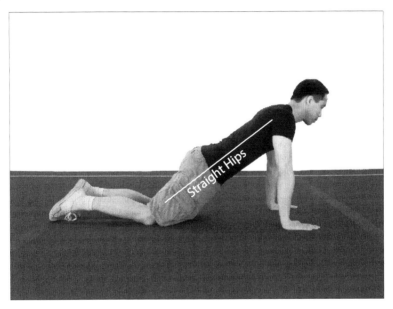

Straight Hips

Basic Progressions

Comments

This exercise gives you a sense of what it will feel like to keep your hips straight under the load of your body weight. You should note the increased stress on your arms as well as the increased contraction necessary from your abs. You may also notice that you are engaging your butt and lower back muscles. However, by bending the knees, the total weight you need to support is reduced, making it easier than a fully extended front plank.

Tips

» Make sure you don't let your hips sag or your back arch downward, especially when you get tired. Keep your abs tight at all times.

Muscles Worked

Front: Pectorals, Front Deltoids, Abdominals, Obliques, Serratus, Hip Flexors, Hip Adductors

Back: Rotator Cuff, Triceps, Trapezius, Lats, Rhomboids, Lower Back, Gluteus Maximus, Hip Abductors

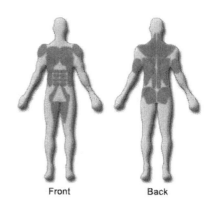

Front   Back

Front Plank

Difficulty: ★★☆☆☆

Directions

Place your hands shoulder-width apart on the ground in front of you and lie prone on the ground in a push-up position. Push up and hold your entire body straight. Your weight will be on your hands and feet. Make sure to keep your shoulders directly over your hands.

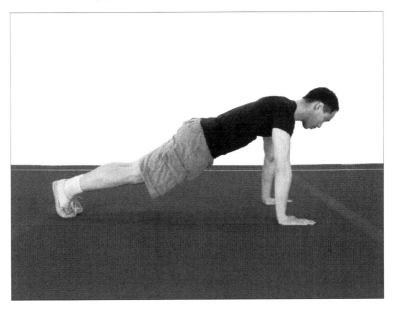

Comments

This is the first fully extended front plank exercise, and it will give your core muscles a great workout. Since it is fully extended, you will be engaging your leg muscles, including the quads and hip flexors. Maintaining this position will also require the antagonistic muscles, such as the hamstrings and glutes, to engage. It may seem easy at first, but as you hold this position for longer periods of time, you may start shaking. This is normal and just indicates that your muscles are getting tired. Eventually, you will develop enough strength for the shaking to go away.

Tips

» Remember to keep your entire body straight. If you find your hips sagging, you can try hollowing your body just a little bit to extend your session by a few seconds. However, you shouldn't move on to the next exercise until you can do this one with a straight body for one full minute.

Muscles Worked

Front: Pectorals, Front Deltoids, Abdominals, Obliques, Serratus, Hip Flexors, Hip Adductors, Quads

Back: Rotator Cuff, Triceps, Trapezius, Lats, Rhomboids, Lower Back, Gluteus Maximus, Hip Abductors, Hamstrings

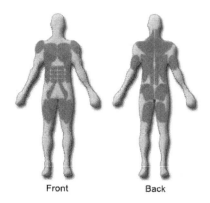

Front   Back

Front Plank: Arms Forward Lv1

Difficulty: ★★☆☆☆

Directions

Place your hands shoulder-width apart on the ground in front of you and lie prone on the ground in a push-up position. Move your hands forward about one foot. Push up and hold your body straight. Your weight will be on your hands and feet. Alternatively, you can start in a front plank position and move your hands forward the appropriate distance.

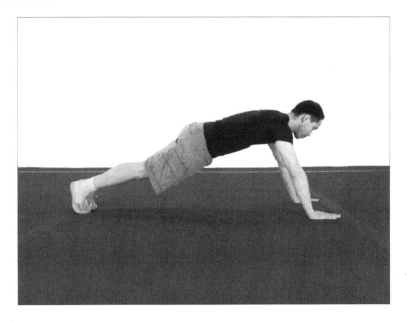

**Basic
Progressions**

Comments

In this branch of the progression, the arms will be moving forward, away from the balance point below your shoulders. This will increase the load on your abs that is required to keep your body straight. This "reverse leveraged" position will also start working more on your *latissimus* muscles.

Tips

» If you find it too difficult at first, you can introduce a slight hollow to your body to help engage the abs better. Be sure not to rely on your lower back muscles more than your abs.

Muscles Worked

Front: Pectorals, Biceps, Abdominals, Obliques, Serratus, Hip Flexors, Hip Adductors, Quads

Back: Rear Deltoids, Rotator Cuff, Triceps, Trapezius, Lats, Rhomboids, Lower Back, Gluteus Maximus, Hip Abductors, Hamstrings

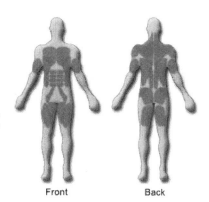

Front   Back

Front Plank: Arms Forward Lv2

Difficulty: ★★★☆☆

Directions

Place your hands shoulder-width apart on the ground in front of you and lie prone on the ground in a push-up position. Move your hands forward about two feet. Push up and hold your body straight. Your weight will be on your hands and feet. Alternatively, you can start in a front plank position and move your hands forward the appropriate distance.

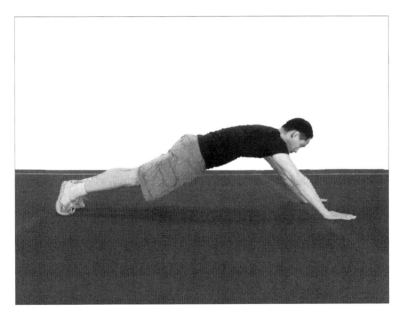

Comments

This exercise increases the load on your abs, lats, and upper chest even more.

Tips

» In this position, your feet and hands may start slipping a bit. If this happens, try doing the exercise on a less slippery floor, or wear some shoes and/or tacky gloves. However, for the ultimate workout, you should rely only on your strength to stop yourself from slipping.

» At this level, you may need to add a slight hollow to your body position so your hips don't sag when you get tired.

Muscles Worked

Front: Pectorals, Biceps, Wrist Flexors, Abdominals, Obliques, Serratus, Hip Flexors, Hip Adductors, Quads

Back: Rear Deltoids, Rotator Cuff, Triceps, Trapezius, Lats, Rhomboids, Lower Back, Gluteus Maximus, Hip Abductors, Hamstrings

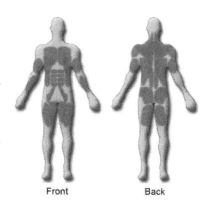

Front   Back

Basic Progressions

Front Plank: Arms Forward Lv3

Difficulty: ★★★★☆

Directions

Place your hands shoulder-width apart on the ground in front of you and lie prone on the ground in a push-up position. Move your hands forward almost as far as you can reach. Push up and hold your body straight. Your weight will be on your hands and feet. Alternatively, you can start in a front plank position and move your hands forward the appropriate distance.

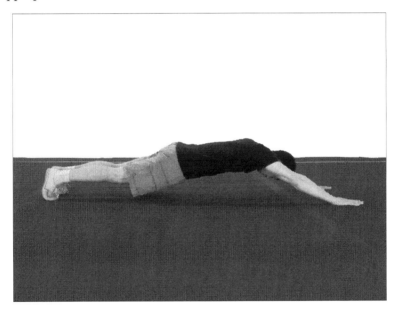

Comments

This is a very difficult exercise and it will work all of the involved muscles very intensely.

Tips

» Be sure to engage your shoulders so that they are pulled into their sockets, not extended out and loose. You will need to push down very hard with your lats and chest muscles at the same time.

» Maintaining a slight hollow will help prevent your lower back from experiencing the majority of the load.

Muscles Worked

Front: Pectorals, Biceps, Wrist Flexors, Abdominals, Obliques, Serratus, Hip Flexors, Hip Adductors, Quads

Back: Rear Deltoids, Rotator Cuff, Triceps, Trapezius, Lats, Rhomboids, Lower Back, Gluteus Maximus, Hip Abductors, Hamstrings

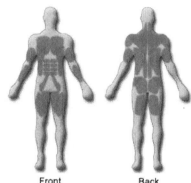

Front   Back

Front Plank: Arms Back Lv1

Difficulty: ★★☆☆☆

Directions

Place your hands shoulder-width apart on the ground in front of you and lie prone on the ground in a push-up position. Move your hands back toward your legs about six inches. Push up and hold your body straight. Your weight will be on your hands and feet, with more of it on your hands. Alternatively, you can start in a front plank position and move your hands backward the appropriate distance.

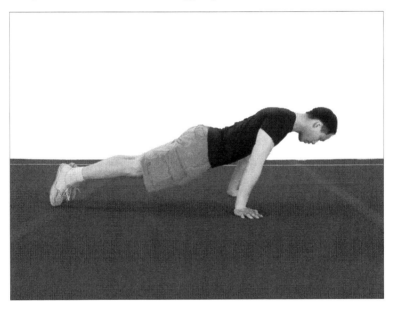

Comments

This branch of the progression will intensify the load on your triceps. It will also start engaging your biceps, since they will be working to keep your elbows from hyperextending. You may notice that these exercises are similar to the Front Planche Leans (see "Chapter 27: Planches"). You can certainly do them the same way, but you don't necessarily need to worry about protracting the shoulders as much here. The goal here is to maximize your arm and chest pushing strength, not the shoulders or the balance.

Tips

» In this and later exercises in this branch, you will be leaning forward so much that you may need to find something to hook your feet onto/over so that you can maintain your balance. This way, you can just focus on the downward pushing component. Of course, if you can do the exercises without any aids, that's even better!

» You may find that your wrists are not flexible enough to keep your fingers facing forward. If that is the case, you can try turning your fingers out to the side until the position is more comfortable.

Muscles Worked

Front: Pectorals, Front Deltoids, Biceps, Abdominals, Obliques, Serratus, Hip Flexors, Hip Adductors, Quads

Back: Rotator Cuff, Triceps, Trapezius, Lats, Rhomboids, Lower Back, Gluteus Maximus, Hip Abductors, Hamstrings

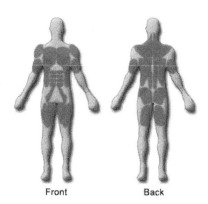

Front   Back

Front Plank: Arms Back Lv2

Difficulty: ★★★☆☆

Directions

Place your hands shoulder-width apart on the ground in front of you and lie prone on the ground in a push-up position. Move your hands back toward your legs so they are just above your waist. Push up and hold your body straight. Your weight will be on your hands and feet, with most of it on the hands. Alternatively, you can start in a front plank position and move your hands backward the appropriate distance.

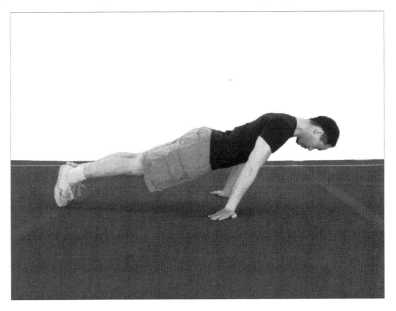

Comments

With so much focus on pushing down and back, you may forget to keep your back straight. Make sure you don't let your hips sag during this exercise, since it is also designed to work on your core.

Tips

» This is a difficult exercise, and it is quite easy to fall forward if you are not strong enough. At first, you can use something to help keep you from falling so you can focus on the downward pushing component. You may also opt to use something soft as a landing cushion in case you do fall.

» You may find it more comfortable for your wrists to turn your hands out to the side.

Muscles Worked

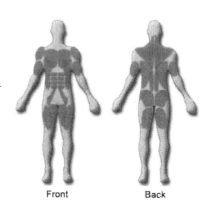

Front: Pectorals, Front Deltoids, Biceps, Abdominals, Obliques, Serratus, Hip Flexors, Hip Adductors, Quads

Back: Rotator Cuff, Triceps, Trapezius, Lats, Rhomboids, Lower Back, Gluteus Maximus, Hip Abductors, Hamstrings

Front   Back

Front Plank: Arms Back Lv3

Difficulty: ★★★★☆

Directions

Place your hands shoulder-width apart on the ground in front of you and lie prone on the ground in a push-up position. Move your hands back toward your legs to just at or slightly below your hips. Push up and hold your body straight. Your weight will be mostly on your hands and just a bit on your feet. Alternatively, you can start in a front plank position and move your hands backward the appropriate distance.

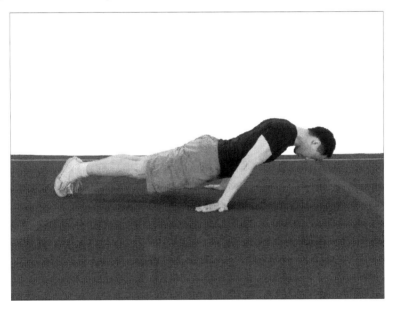

Comments

This is an extremely difficult exercise and you will most likely fall forward unless you have something in place to keep you from doing so, such as an object to hook your feet onto. You will also likely need to turn your hands so that your fingers are pointing toward your feet.

Tips

» Since this is a difficult exercise, it is quite easy to fall forward, especially when you get tired. At first, you can use something to help keep you from falling so you can focus on the downward pushing component. You may also opt to use something soft as a landing cushion in case you do fall.

» You may find it more comfortable for your wrists to turn your hands out to the side.

Muscles Worked

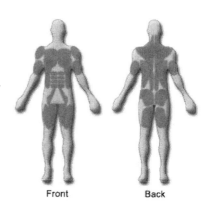

Front: Pectorals, Front Deltoids, Biceps, Abdominals, Obliques, Serratus, Hip Flexors, Hip Adductors, Quads

Back: Rotator Cuff, Triceps, Trapezius, Lats, Rhomboids, Lower Back, Gluteus Maximus, Hip Abductors, Hamstrings

Front   Back

Front Plank: Arms Side Lv1

Difficulty: ★★☆☆☆

Directions

Place your hands shoulder-width apart on the ground in front of you and lie prone on the ground in a push-up position. Move each hand about one foot out to the side. Push up and hold your body straight. Your weight will be on your hands and feet. Alternatively, you can start in a front plank position and move your hands sideways the appropriate distance.

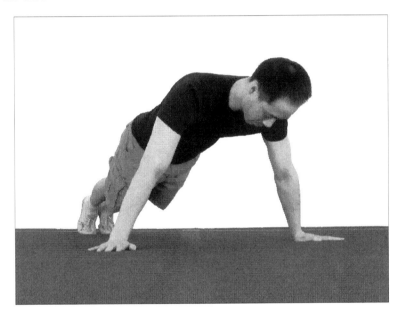

Comments

This branch of the progression starts working on wide arm pushing strength, which will give your chest muscles a great workout. Since the hands are still in line with the shoulders, balance should not be an issue here.

Tips

> » You may find it easier to turn your hands so that your fingers are facing outward.

» If you want to work on your biceps as well, you can rotate your elbows so that your elbow pits point toward the ground. This will require you to internally rotate your shoulders. To keep your shoulders safe, be sure to engage your shoulder muscles so that the shoulders are pulled down into their sockets. Use your back muscles to help maintain this shoulder position.

Muscles Worked

Front: Pectorals, Front Deltoids, Biceps, Abdominals, Obliques, Serratus, Hip Flexors, Hip Adductors, Quads

Back: Rotator Cuff, Triceps, Trapezius, Lats, Rhomboids, Lower Back, Gluteus Maximus, Hip Abductors, Hamstrings

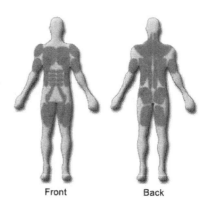

Front   Back

Front Plank: Arms Side Lv2

Difficulty: ★★★☆☆

Directions

Place your hands shoulder-width apart on the ground in front of you and lie prone on the ground in a push-up position. Move each hand about two and a half feet out to the side. Push up and hold your body straight. Your weight will be on your hands and feet. Alternatively, you can start in a front plank position and move your hands sideways the appropriate distance.

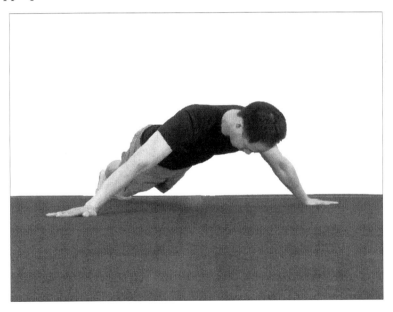

Comments

This exercise is similar to the previous one but provides a more intense workout. Since the hands are still in line with the shoulders, balance should not be an issue here.

Tips

» You may find it easier to turn your hands so that your fingers are facing outward.

» If you want to work on your biceps as well, you can rotate your elbows so that your elbow pits point toward the ground. This will require you to internally rotate your shoulders. To keep your shoulders safe, be sure to engage your shoulder muscles so that the shoulders are pulled down into their sockets. Use your back muscles to help maintain the shoulder position.

Muscles Worked

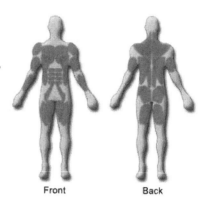

Front

Back

Front: Pectorals, Front Deltoids, Biceps, Wrist Flexors, Abdominals, Obliques, Serratus, Hip Flexors, Hip Adductors, Quads

Back: Rotator Cuff, Triceps, Trapezius, Lats, Rhomboids, Lower Back, Gluteus Maximus, Hip Abductors, Hamstrings

Front Plank: Arms Side Lv3

Difficulty: ★★★★☆

Directions

Place your hands shoulder-width apart on the ground in front of you and lie prone on the ground in a push-up position. Move your hands out to the side almost as far as you can reach. Push up and hold your body straight. Your weight will be on your hands and feet. Alternatively, you can start in a front plank position and move your hands sideways the appropriate distance.

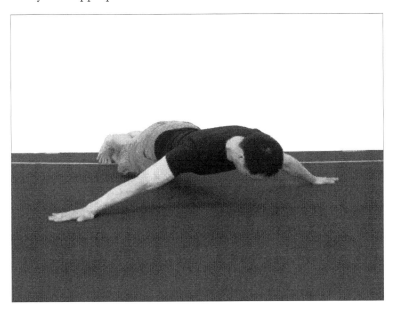

Comments

This exercise is the most intense in this branch of the progression. It feels similar to the straight-arm butterfly movement usually performed with dumbbells. However, holding this "reverse leveraged" position for a full minute is quite difficult. Since the hands are still in line with the shoulders, balance should not be an issue here.

Tips

»   You may find it easier to turn your hands so that your fingers are facing outward.

» If you want to work on your biceps as well, you can rotate your elbows so that your elbow pits point toward the ground. This will require you to internally rotate your shoulders. To keep your shoulders safe, be sure to engage your shoulder muscles so that the shoulders are pulled down into their sockets. Use your back muscles to help maintain the shoulder position.

Muscles Worked

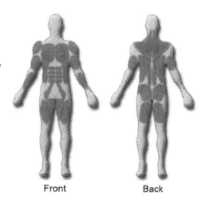

Front: Pectorals, Front Deltoids, Biceps, Wrist Flexors, Abdominals, Obliques, Serratus, Hip Flexors, Hip Adductors, Quads

Back: Rotator Cuff, Triceps, Trapezius, Lats, Rhomboids, Lower Back, Gluteus Maximus, Hip Abductors, Hamstrings

Front   Back

19

Back Planks

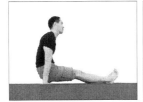 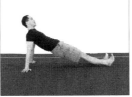 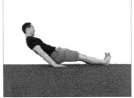

| Beginner | Mid-Level | Advanced |

The Back Plank Progression works on your core muscles from a different direction than the Front Plank Progression. As the name implies, it focuses more strongly on the back muscles, but it also works on the glutes, triceps, and rear shoulders. These exercises will help with shoulder flexibility, especially the Arms Back variation. Balance is generally not an issue, except for in the most advanced exercises.

The back plank position looks similar to the front plank, except your body is facing up. Once you get to the fully extended back planks, the goal is to keep the body as straight as possible.

Like the front plank, sagging at the hips will reduce the benefits gained from this exercise and will hinder progress to the advanced exercises. However, unlike the front plank, sagging generally will not increase the load on your abdominal muscles, since your body naturally bends in that direction. Instead, your body will just end up in a hollow position. In the worst case scenario, you will find yourself sitting back down on the ground. You should avoid over-arching your back as that can lead to excessive strain on the lower back.

Equipment Needed

Floor space

These exercises are usually performed on the floor, but you can also use bar-type handles or even low hanging rings. If you have wrist problems, it may be difficult for you to support your weight with your hands on the floor. In this case, you can try using push-up handles. These handles will allow you to keep your wrists in a neutral position. Working with rings will make the exercises more difficult, but your stabilizing muscles will develop faster. This is beneficial to your shoulder joints, since they will become stronger and more resistant to injury.

General Notes

If you have rotator cuff issues, the back plank exercises are also a good way to strengthen the muscles around the shoulder. Since these exercises are static, you will be better able to focus on muscle recruitment and body position. You will also run a lower chance of irritating old or nagging injuries compared to dynamic exercises. In addition, you will develop a better feel for how the muscles in your body work. This is critical to improving athletic ability and reducing risk of injury in the future.

Exercise Map

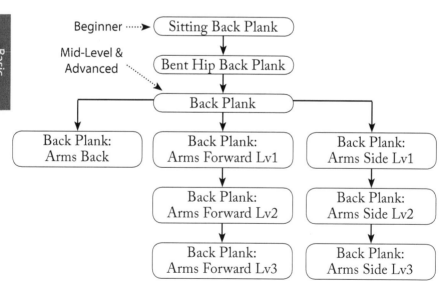

Sitting Back Plank

Difficulty: ★☆☆☆☆

Directions

Place your hands on the floor beside your butt. Push up and lift your butt off the ground. Keep your feet on the ground.

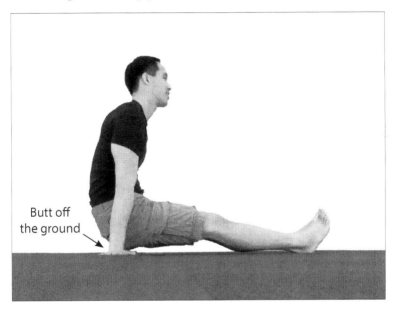

Butt off the ground

Comments

This exercise allows you to work on your downward pushing strength without worrying about core strength. Make sure to keep your shoulders pressed down so that you can get maximum lift.

Basic Progressions

Sitting Back Plank

Muscles Worked

Front: Pectorals, Abdominals, Obliques

Back: Rotator Cuff, Triceps, Trapezius, Lats, Rhomboids

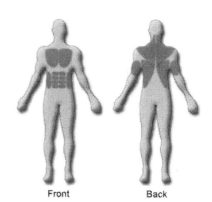

Front   Back

Bent Hip Plank

Difficulty: ★☆☆☆☆

Directions

Place your hands on the floor beside or slightly behind you. Push up, lifting your butt off the ground, and slide your feet forward until your legs and upper body form a 135-degree angle at the hip. Keep your feet on the ground and make sure your shoulders are directly over your hands.

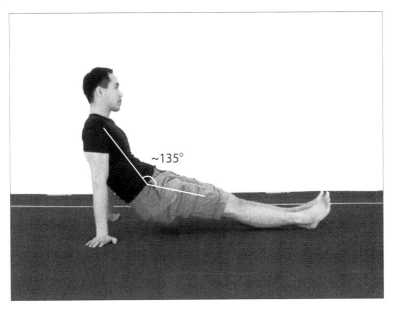

~135°

Comments

This exercise starts engaging the core muscles, especially the back and glutes.

Tips

 » You can try squeezing your legs together to target the leg adductors. This will also increase intensity for the glutes.

Bent Hip Plank

Muscles Worked

Front: Pectorals, Abdominals, Obliques, Serratus

Back: Rear Deltoids, Rotator Cuff, Triceps, Trapezius, Lats, Rhomboids, Lower Back, Gluteus Maximus, Hamstrings

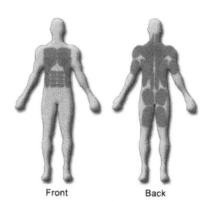

Front   Back

Back Plank

Difficulty: ★⯪☆☆☆

Directions

Place your hands on the floor beside or slightly behind you. Push up, lifting your butt off the ground, and slide your feet forward until your legs and upper body are in a straight line. Keep your feet on the ground and make sure your shoulders are directly over your hands.

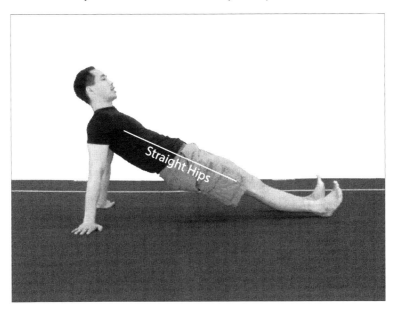

Comments

This is the first exercise in this progression to reach the fully extended position. You will need to engage your hamstrings in addition to your glutes and core muscles to maintain proper form. Maintaining this position will also require you to engage the antagonistic muscles, such as the quads. Like the fully extended front plank, it may seem easy at first, but as you hold the position for longer periods of time, you may start shaking. This is normal and indicates that your muscles are getting tired. Eventually, you will develop enough strength and the shaking will go away.

Tips

> » Remember to keep your entire body straight. If you find your hips sagging, think about pushing your hips up and focus on contracting your glutes and lower back more.

> » You can try squeezing your legs together to target the leg adductors. This will also increase intensity for the glutes.

Muscles Worked

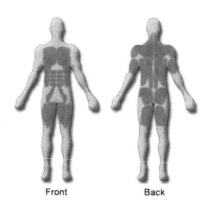

Front   Back

Front: Pectorals, Abdominals, Obliques, Serratus, Hip Flexors, Hip Adductors, Quads

Back: Rear Deltoids, Rotator Cuff, Triceps, Trapezius, Lats, Rhomboids, Lower Back, Gluteus Maximus, Hip Abductors, Hamstrings

Back Plank: Arms Back

Difficulty: ★★☆☆☆

Directions

Place your hands on the floor beside and slightly behind you. Push up, lifting your butt off the ground, and slide your feet forward until your legs and upper body are in a straight line. Make sure you slide forward enough so that your shoulders are about a foot in front of your hands.

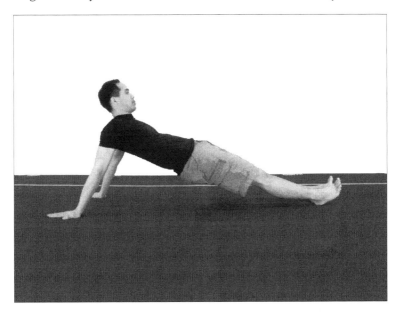

Comments

The amount you can slide forward will likely be limited by your shoulder flexibility. Move forward enough to feel a good stretch in the shoulders, but not to the point where they hurt. This position will engage your upper back in a different way than the regular back plank.

Tips

» Remember to keep your entire body straight. If you find your hips sagging, think about pushing your hips up and focus on contracting your glutes and lower back more.

Basic Progressions

» You can try squeezing your legs together to target the leg adductors. This will also increase intensity for the glutes.

Muscles Worked

Front: Pectorals, Front Deltoids, Biceps, Wrist Flexors, Abdominals, Obliques, Serratus, Hip Flexors, Hip Adductors, Quads

Back: Rear Deltoids, Rotator Cuff, Triceps, Trapezius, Lats, Rhomboids, Lower Back, Gluteus Maximus, Hip Abductors, Hamstrings

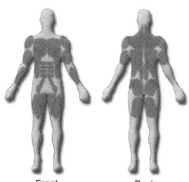

Front   Back

Back Plank: Arms Forward Lv1

Difficulty: ★★☆☆☆

Directions

Place your hands on the floor beside you and slightly in front of your hips. Push up, lifting your butt off the ground and into the back plank position. Keeping your legs and upper body in a straight line, lean backward and let your feet slide until your shoulders are about one foot behind your hands.

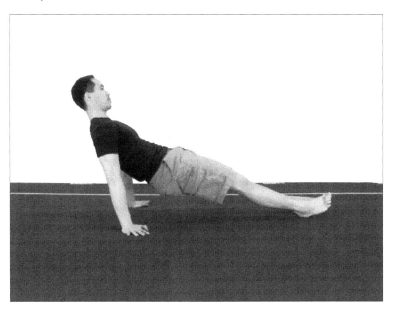

Comments

This branch of the progression adds reverse leverage, which increases the work your upper back muscles and glutes have to do. It will also be harder to keep your body in a straight line.

Tips

> » Really focus on pushing the hips up toward the ceiling (or sky) and contract your lower back, glutes, and hamstrings to help maintain the position. Squeezing your legs together will also engage your leg adductors, allowing you to work additional muscles during this exercise.

Back Plank: Arms Forward Lv1

Muscles Worked

Front: Pectorals, Front Deltoids, Wrist Flexors, Abdominals, Obliques, Serratus, Hip Flexors, Hip Adductors, Quads

Back: Rear Deltoids, Rotator Cuff, Triceps, Trapezius, Lats, Rhomboids, Lower Back, Gluteus Maximus, Hip Abductors, Hamstrings

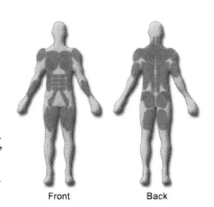

Front   Back

Basic Progressions

Back Plank: Arms Forward Lv2

Difficulty: ★★★☆☆

Directions

Place your hands on the floor beside you and slightly in front of your hips. Push up, lifting your butt off the ground and into the back plank position. Keeping your legs and upper body in a straight line, lean backward and let your feet slide until your waist is above your hands.

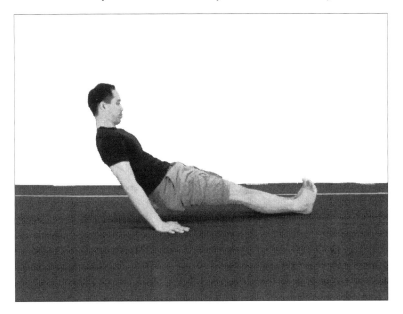

Comments

This is a very difficult exercise due to the increased amount of reverse leverage. Make sure to keep your arms straight. It will also require additional strength to maintain your balance. Your triceps and rear shoulder muscles will get an intense workout from this exercise.

Tips

» If you have difficulty maintaining balance, you can try hooking your feet onto something to prevent them from sliding back.

» At this level, unless you have very flexible wrists, you will probably need to turn your hands out to the sides, or have them face forward.

Muscles Worked

Front: Pectorals, Front Deltoids, Wrist Flexors, Abdominals, Obliques, Serratus, Hip Flexors, Hip Adductors, Quads

Back: Rear Deltoids, Rotator Cuff, Triceps, Trapezius, Lats, Rhomboids, Lower Back, Gluteus Maximus, Hip Abductors, Hamstrings

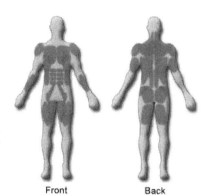

Front   Back

Back Plank: Arms Forward Lv3

Difficulty: ★★★★☆

Directions

Place your hands on the floor beside you and slightly in front of your hips. Push up, lifting your butt off the ground and into the back plank position. Keeping your legs and upper body in a straight line, lean backward and let your feet slide until your hands are below or slightly past your hips.

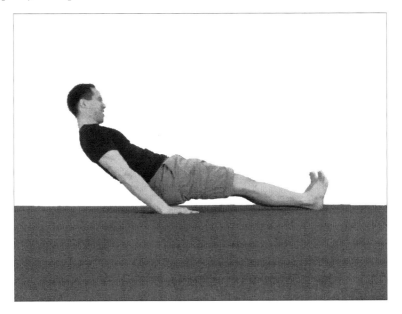

Comments

This is an extremely difficult exercise. Not only is the reverse leverage increased dramatically, balance comes into play here as well.

Tips

» You will likely need to hook your feet onto something to prevent you from falling back. This way, you can focus on your body position and pressing down as hard as you can. You will need to turn your hands out to the side or front for this exercise.

Back Plank: Arms Forward Lv3

Muscles Worked

Front: Pectorals, Front Deltoids, Wrist Flexors, Abdominals, Obliques, Serratus, Hip Flexors, Hip Adductors, Quads

Back: Rear Deltoids, Rotator Cuff, Triceps, Trapezius, Lats, Rhomboids, Lower Back, Gluteus Maximus, Hip Abductors, Hamstrings

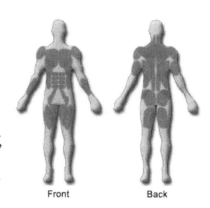

Front   Back

Back Plank: Arms Side Lv1

Difficulty: ★★☆☆☆

Directions

Place your hands on the floor beside you, a foot away to each side. Push up, lifting your butt off the ground, and slide your feet forward until your legs and upper body are in a straight line. Your hands and shoulders should all be in the same vertical plane.

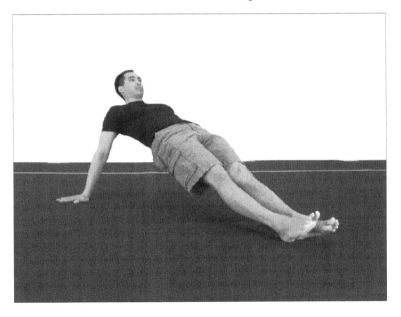

Comments

This branch of the progression adds reverse leverage, which increases the work on your upper back muscles.

Tips

» Focus on keeping the hips pushed up when you perform this exercise. Squeezing your legs together will also target your leg adductors.

Back Plank: Arms Side Lv1

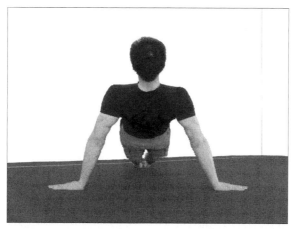

Alternate View

Muscles Worked

Front: Pectorals, Front Deltoids, Biceps, Wrist Flexors, Abdominals, Obliques, Serratus, Hip Flexors, Hip Adductors, Quads

Back: Rear Deltoids, Rotator Cuff, Triceps, Trapezius, Lats, Rhomboids, Lower Back, Gluteus Maximus, Hip Abductors, Hamstrings

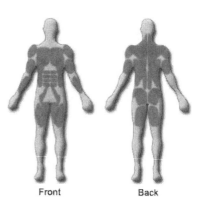

Front   Back

Back Plank: Arms Side Lv2

Difficulty: ★★★☆☆

Directions

Place your hands on the floor beside you, about two to two-and-a-half feet away to each side. Push up, lifting your butt off the ground, and slide your feet forward until your legs and upper body are in a straight line. Your hands and shoulders should all be in the same vertical plane.

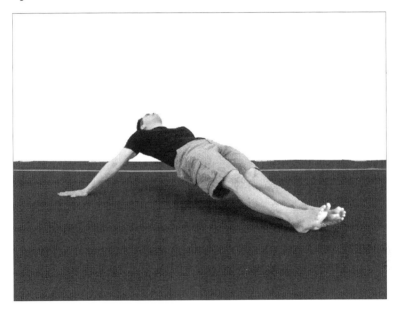

Comments

This exercise builds on the previous one by increasing reverse leverage. You will need to contract all of your upper back muscles intensely to maintain this position.

Tips

» It will help to squeeze your shoulder blades together.

» Focus on keeping the hips pushed up when you perform this exercise. Squeezing your legs together will also target your leg adductors.

Back Plank: Arms Side Lv2

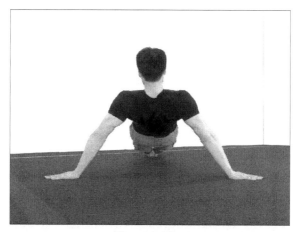

Alternate View

Muscles Worked

Front: Pectorals, Front Deltoids, Biceps, Wrist Flexors, Abdominals, Obliques, Serratus, Hip Flexors, Hip Adductors, Quads

Back: Rear Deltoids, Rotator Cuff, Triceps, Trapezius, Lats, Rhomboids, Lower Back, Gluteus Maximus, Hip Abductors, Hamstrings

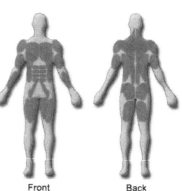

Front   Back

Back Plank: Arms Side Lv3

Difficulty: ★★★★☆

Directions

While lying on your back, place your hands on the floor beside you, almost as far as you can reach to each side. Push up, lifting your butt off the ground, and slide your feet forward until your legs and upper body are in a straight line. Your hands and shoulders should all be in the same vertical plane.

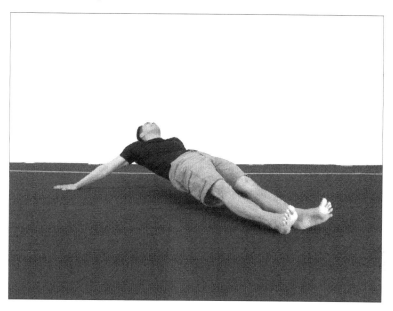

Comments

This exercise is extremely difficult and will build immense back strength.

Tips

» Be sure to keep your shoulder blades squeezed together and arms straight throughout the entire exercise.

» Focus on keeping your hips pushed up when you perform this exercise. Squeezing your legs together will also target your leg adductors.

Back Plank: Arms Side Lv3

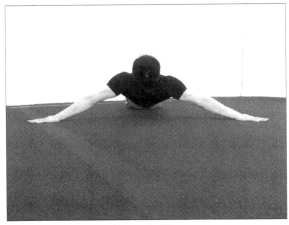

Alternate View

Muscles Worked

Front: Pectorals, Front Deltoids, Biceps, Wrist Flexors, Abdominals, Obliques, Serratus, Hip Flexors, Hip Adductors, Quads

Back: Rear Deltoids, Rotator Cuff, Triceps, Trapezius, Lats, Rhomboids, Lower Back, Gluteus Maximus, Hip Abductors, Hamstrings

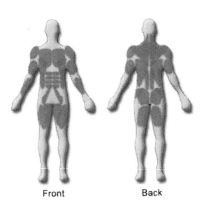

Front   Back

Basic
Progressions

20

Side Planks

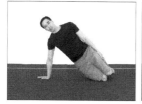
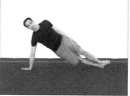
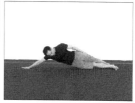

Beginner   Mid-Level   Advanced

The Side Plank Progression develops the often-neglected oblique muscles of the core. Our bodies can bend and twist in many directions at the waist, so we need to make sure that our side-to-side movements are just as strong as the forward-backward movements. The earlier exercises will focus mainly on core strength, while the advanced exercises will also include intense work on the lats.

These exercises involve balancing on two points (one hand and one foot). Therefore, they may be more difficult until your muscles develop enough strength to maintain good balance. When you get to the advanced exercises, you will find that there is tremendous emphasis on strength. At this point, you may find it helpful to separate your feet a little bit so that you can work with a more stable base.

Since these exercises are one-sided, they work the muscles on one side of your body differently than the other side. It is best to work both sides of your body equally so that you minimize the chances of developing muscle imbalances. Therefore, it is recommended that you do the same number of seconds of an exercise on each side. You can let the total time for both sides add up to one minute, or you can complete an entire minute on each side. Of course, doing the latter will help you progress faster.

There are several variations you can use that will work your leg muscles in even more ways. One variation is to use just the bottom leg for support. This way, you can raise the top leg, which is no longer supporting any weight, up to a horizontal position. This enables you to work on the abductor muscles on both hips at the same time. Note that this may make it more difficult to maintain your balance, so you will need to decide if you are ready for this variation or not.

Another variation is to use just the top leg to support your body in the side plank position. The bottom leg should then be lifted up as high as it can go, either in front of or behind the support leg. This enables you to work on the adductors of both legs at the same time.

Equipment Needed

Floor Space

These exercises are usually performed on the floor, but you can also use bar-type handles or even low hanging rings. If you have wrist problems, it may be difficult for you to support your weight with your hands on the floor. In this case, you can try using push-up handles. These handles will allow you to keep your wrists in a neutral position. Working with rings will make the exercises more difficult, but your stabilizing muscles will develop faster. This is beneficial to your shoulder joints, since they will become stronger and more resistant to injury.

Basic
Progressions

Exercise Map

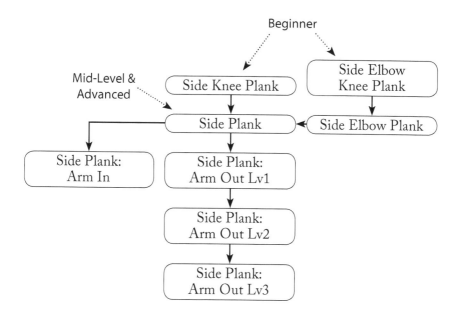

Basic
Progressions

Side Knee Plank

Difficulty: ★☆☆☆☆

Directions

Place one hand on the ground to the side of your body. Keeping your knees bent and on the ground, lift your butt up so that your thighs and upper body are in a straight line. Your hand should be directly below your shoulder.

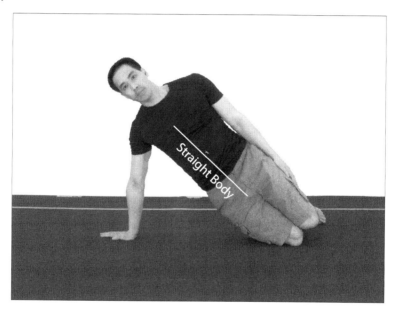

Comments

This exercise will help you get used to engaging the oblique muscles in your core, as well as your hip abductors.

Tips

» Be sure to engage your shoulder muscles by pressing the shoulder down, away from your ears. This will allow you to utilize the bigger muscles in your upper body.

Side Knee Plank

Muscles Worked

Front: Pectorals, Front Deltoids, Abdominals, Obliques, Serratus, Hip Flexors, Hip Adductors, Quads

Back: Rear Deltoids, Rotator Cuff, Triceps, Trapezius, Lats, Rhomboids, Lower Back, Gluteus Maximus, Hip Abductors, Hamstrings

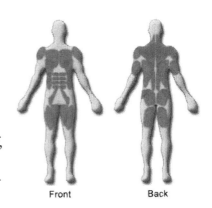

Front   Back

Side Plank

Difficulty: ★☆☆☆☆

Directions

Place one hand on the ground to the side of your body. Keeping your legs straight and feet on the ground, lift your butt up so that your legs and upper body are in a straight line. Your hand should be directly below your shoulder.

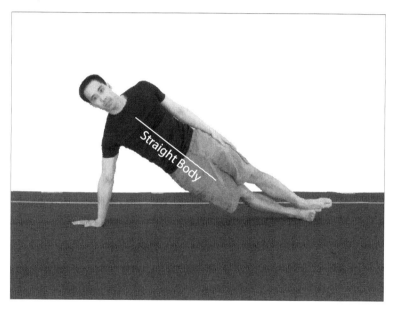

Comments

This is the full side plank position. You will need to press down with your feet and engage your hip abductors in order to maintain this position. Even though you are on your side, you may need to engage your front and back core muscles as well as your upper torso muscles to help maintain your balance. This is especially important when you get tired. It may seem easy at first, but as you hold the position for longer periods of time, you may start shaking. This is normal, and it just indicates that your muscles are getting tired. Eventually, you will develop enough strength, and the shaking will go away. Again, remember to keep your whole body straight the entire time.

Basic
Progressions

Tips

» If needed, you can separate your feet a bit for additional stability.

Variations

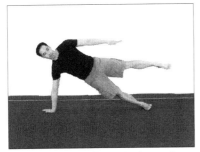 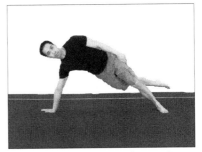

Top Arm and Leg Horizontal   *Bottom Leg Crossed in Back*

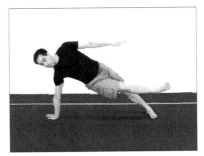

Bottom Leg Crossed in Front

Muscles Worked

Front: Pectorals, Front Deltoids, Abdominals, Obliques, Serratus, Hip Flexors, Hip Adductors, Quads

Back: Rear Deltoids, Rotator Cuff, Triceps, Trapezius, Lats, Rhomboids, Lower Back, Gluteus Maximus, Hip Abductors, Hamstrings

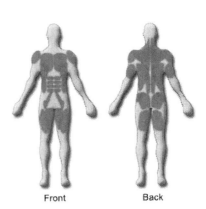

Front   Back

Side Plank: Arm Out Lv1

Difficulty: ★★☆☆☆

Directions

Place one hand on the ground to the side of your body, a foot further to the side than usual. Keeping your legs straight and feet on the ground, lift your butt up so that your legs and upper body are in a straight line.

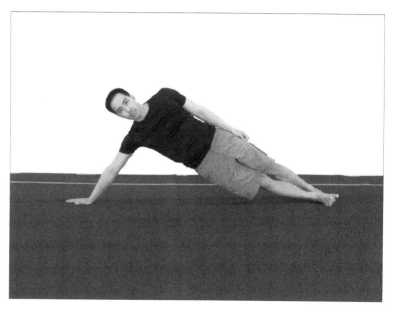

Comments

This exercise introduces some reverse leverage, making it more difficult than the full side plank. You will need to engage the lats more in order to maintain this position. You may also find yourself working harder to maintain your balance.

Tips

» If needed, you can separate your feet a bit for additional stability.

» If you are on a slick surface, you may find it even more difficult to perform this exercise. If needed, you can try using some aids that make the surface less slippery (e.g. shoes). However, relying only on your muscles will give you better results more quickly.

Muscles Worked

Front: Pectorals, Front Deltoids, Biceps, Wrist Flexors, Abdominals, Obliques, Serratus, Hip Flexors, Hip Adductors, Quads

Back: Rear Deltoids, Rotator Cuff, Triceps, Trapezius, Lats, Rhomboids, Lower Back, Gluteus Maximus, Hip Abductors, Hamstrings

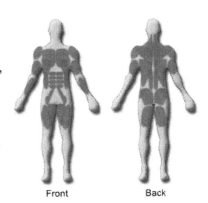

Front   Back

Side Plank: Arm Out Lv2

Difficulty: ★★★☆☆

Directions

Place one hand on the ground to the side of your body, about two to two-and-a-half feet further out than usual. Keeping your legs straight and feet on the ground, lift your butt up so that your legs and upper body are in a straight line.

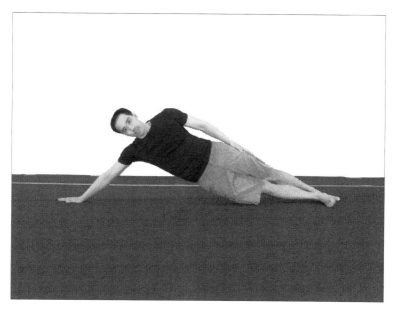

Comments

This exercise increases reverse leverage significantly. You will need to engage all of your core muscles as well as your upper back and chest muscles to maintain this position.

Tips

»   If needed, you can separate your feet a bit for additional stability.

»   You may also want to rotate the elbow of your support arm so that the elbow pit faces the ground. This will allow you to engage your biceps to help maintain a straight support arm.

» Remember to keep the shoulder pressed down, especially if you turn your elbows to engage the biceps. Doing so will help protect your shoulder joint and work on the rotator cuff muscles even more.

» At this level, you may start slipping more, depending on the surface you are exercising on. If that is the case, you can use aids to help reduce the amount of slippage. However, if you are strong enough, it is more effective to rely on your muscles to maintain the position.

Muscles Worked

Front: Pectorals, Front Deltoids, Biceps, Wrist Flexors, Abdominals, Obliques, Serratus, Hip Flexors, Hip Adductors, Quads

Back: Rear Deltoids, Rotator Cuff, Triceps, Trapezius, Lats, Rhomboids, Lower Back, Gluteus Maximus, Hip Abductors, Hamstrings

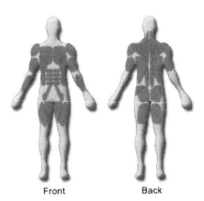

Front   Back

Side Plank: Arm Out Lv3

Difficulty: ★★★★☆

Directions

Lie down on your side. Place the hand on the side closest to the ground up above your head, almost as far as you can reach. Keeping your legs straight and feet on the ground, lift your butt up so that your legs and upper body are in a straight line.

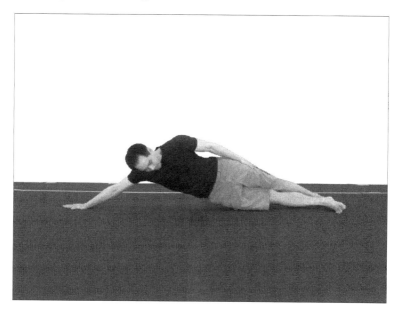

Comments

This exercise requires a lot of strength since your body is in such an extended position. You will likely need to rotate the elbow of your support arm so that the elbow pit faces the ground. This will help you maintain a stronger straight support arm.

Tips

>> If needed, you can separate your feet a bit for additional stability.

>> This is a very difficult exercise, and you may need to use your free hand to help push your body up when getting into the position.

Side Plank: Arm Out Lv3

Muscles Worked

Front: Pectorals, Front Deltoids, Biceps, Wrist Flexors, Abdominals, Obliques, Serratus, Hip Flexors, Hip Adductors, Quads

Back: Rear Deltoids, Rotator Cuff, Triceps, Trapezius, Lats, Rhomboids, Lower Back, Gluteus Maximus, Hip Abductors, Hamstrings

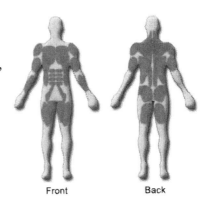

Front   Back

Side Plank: Arm In

Difficulty: ★★☆☆☆

Directions

Place one hand on the ground to the side of your body, about a foot closer to you than usual. Keeping your legs straight and feet on the ground, lift up your butt so that your legs and upper body are in a straight line. Your hand should be directly below your lower chest area.

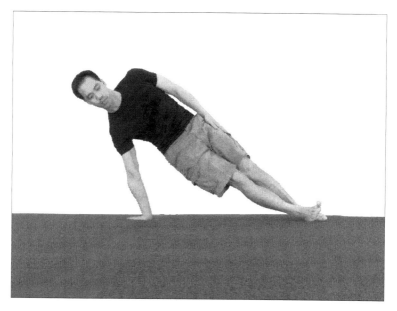

Comments

This exercise is difficult due to the positioning of the hand and wrist. The amount of reverse leverage you can achieve may also be limited by your wrist flexibility. Go only as far as comfortable, not to the point of pain. This exercise will also work on your deltoid muscles due to the nature of the reverse leverage.

Tips

» If your feel a lot of stress in your wrist, you can try pointing your fingers to the front or back.

Side Plank: Arm In

Muscles Worked

Front: Pectorals, Front Deltoids, Wrist Flexors, Abdominals, Obliques, Serratus, Hip Flexors, Hip Adductors, Quads

Back: Rear Deltoids, Rotator Cuff, Triceps, Trapezius, Lats, Rhomboids, Lower Back, Gluteus Maximus, Hip Abductors, Hamstrings

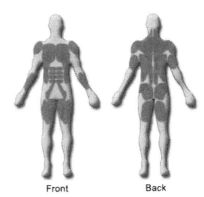

Front   Back

Alternative Start to Progression

Side Elbow Knee Plank

Difficulty: ★☆☆☆☆

Directions

Place one elbow on the ground to the side of your body. Keeping your knees bent and on the ground, lift your butt up so that your thighs and upper body are in a straight line. Your elbow should be directly below your shoulder.

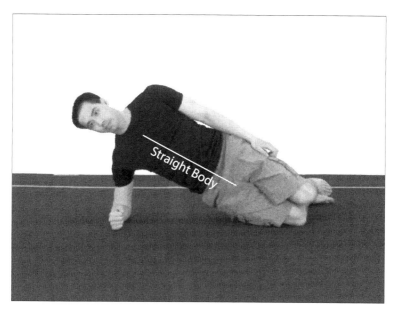

Straight Body

Comments

Technically, this exercise works your core muscles more than the straight arm version. However, with the knees bent, the difference may not be noticeable. The main difference is that you will not need as much arm strength here, since your weight is supported by your elbow. Therefore, this is a good exercise to start with if you lack the strength to perform the straight arm version.

Side Elbow Knee Plank

Muscles Worked

Front: Pectorals, Front Deltoids, Abdominals, Obliques, Serratus, Hip Flexors, Hip Adductors, Quads

Back: Rear Deltoids, Rotator Cuff, Triceps, Trapezius, Lats, Rhomboids, Lower Back, Gluteus Maximus, Hip Abductors, Hamstrings

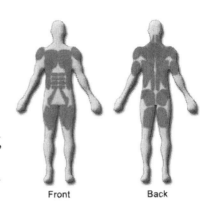

Front   Back

Basic Progressions

Side Elbow Plank

Difficulty: ★☆☆☆☆

Directions

Place one elbow on the ground to the side of your body. Keeping your legs straight and feet on the ground, lift your butt up so that your legs and upper body are in a straight line. Your elbow should be directly below your shoulder.

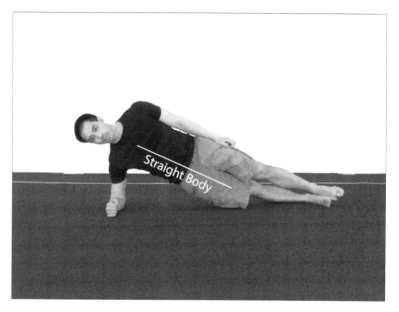

Straight Body

Comments

Like the previous exercise using an elbow support, this will work on the core muscles more than the straight arm version. Again, you will not need to worry about arm strength as much due to the bent elbow position. Once you have mastered this exercise, you should move onto the fully extended side plank with a straight arm support. This way, you will be able to progress to the advanced exercises.

Basic
Progressions

Side Elbow Plank

Muscles Worked

Front: Pectorals, Front Deltoids, Abdominals, Obliques, Serratus, Hip Flexors, Hip Adductors, Quads

Back: Rear Deltoids, Rotator Cuff, Triceps, Trapezius, Lats, Rhomboids, Lower Back, Gluteus Maximus, Hip Abductors, Hamstrings

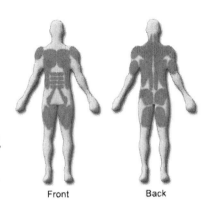

Front   Back

21

Squats

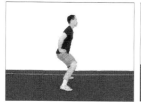 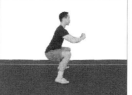 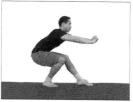

Beginner   Mid-Level   Advanced

The Squat Progression focuses mainly on muscles from the waist down. These exercises will develop strong, balanced leg muscles that can help with knee and hip joint issues. They will also help improve your sense of balance, which can reduce your risk of falls and injury. If you have difficulty with walking and mobility, these exercises can help improve your ability to move around.

When doing any leg-based exercise, balance can always contribute to the difficulty of the exercise. It is important to develop the necessary strength to perform the exercise before focusing on maintaining balance. Therefore, if you find yourself needing some help to balance yourself during an exercise, it's okay to hold on to a support such as a table, chair, wall, or some other stable object. As you get stronger, the exercise will become easier, and you can rely less on the support. Eventually, you will be able to do the exercise without any support. At that point, you can focus mostly on improving your sense of balance, which will work wonders on all of the involved muscles.

If you master an exercise and find the next exercise too difficult to hold for even five seconds, you can temporarily use your hands to push lightly on a nearby support. Make sure you only push enough so that you are just able to do the exercise. This way, you can make sure you are working the intended muscles as much as possible, and not your upper body. As you get stronger, you will be able to stop using your hands for aid.

Equipment Needed

Floor Space
Support for balance, such as a chair or wall (optional)

Exercise Map

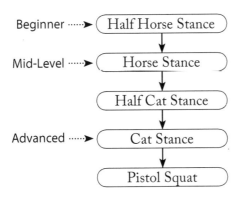

Half Horse Stance

Difficulty: ★☆☆☆☆

Directions

Stand with your feet slightly wider than shoulder-width apart. Keeping your back straight and as vertical as you can, bend your knees to a 135-degree angle. You can place your hands at your sides, or if needed, out to the sides or in front to help with balance. Keep your feet pointing forward and as parallel to each other as possible.

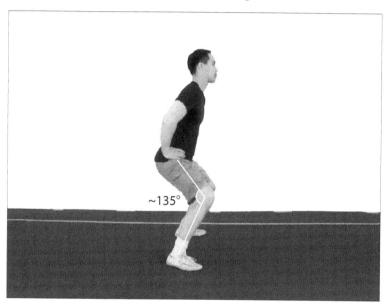

Basic
Progressions

Comments

While this may seem easy for some people, it can become quite tiring as you approach the one-minute mark. Be sure to keep your back straight and upright. Do not slouch or bend forward at the waist. This will force you to engage your core muscles (abs and lower back).

Half Horse Stance

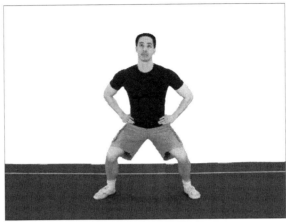

Alternate View

Muscles Worked

Front: Abdominals, Obliques, Hip Adductors, Quads

Back: Lower Back, Gluteus Maximus, Hip Abductors, Hamstrings

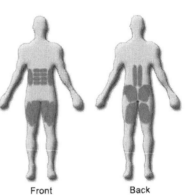

Front   Back

Horse Stance

Difficulty: ★⯪☆☆☆

Directions

Stand with your feet about twice your shoulder-width apart. Keeping your back straight and as vertical as possible, bend your knees until your thighs are parallel to the ground. You can place your hands at your sides, or if needed, out to the sides or in front to help with balance. Keep your feet pointing forward as much as possible, instead of out to the sides.

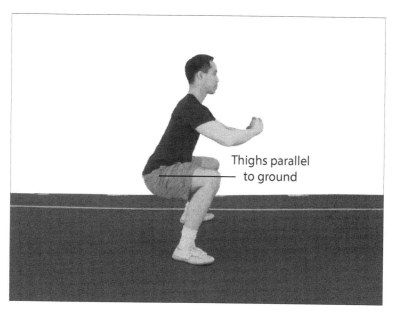

Thighs parallel to ground

Comments

This exercise can quickly tire your thighs, and it is normal for your quads to feel the majority of the effort. Be sure to keep your back straight and as vertical as you can. This will force you to engage your core muscles. By keeping your feet pointing forward, you will better engage your hip adductor muscles, which are critical to maintaining knee joint stability and general mobility.

Tips

» If you can't get your thighs completely parallel to the ground at first, get as close as you can. As you get stronger, you'll eventually be able to reach the parallel position.

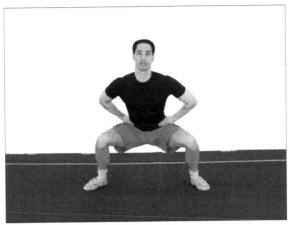

Alternate View

Muscles Worked

Front: Abdominals, Obliques, Hip Adductors, Quads

Back: Lower Back, Gluteus Maximus, Hip Abductors, Hamstrings

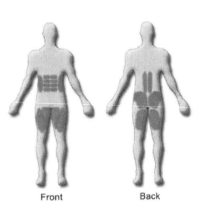

Front   Back

Basic
Progressions

Half Cat Stance

Difficulty: ★★☆☆☆

Directions

Stand with all of your weight on one leg. Keeping your back as upright as possible, bend the supporting knee to a 135-degree angle. Let the foot of the free leg touch the ground lightly, making sure it does not support any of your weight.

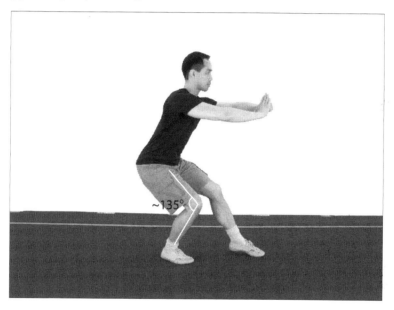

Comments

This exercise will prepare you for more advanced exercises, which are all single-leg standing exercises. Be sure to keep the heel of the supporting foot down. This will give you a bigger support base, which improves stability. Remember that the front foot should not support any of your weight.

Tips

» If you need help with balance, you can touch or hold on to something stable, such as a table or wall. However, don't use it to lighten the load on your target muscles.

» Your free foot may also occasionally press against the floor to help with your balance. As you get stronger, try to avoid doing this so you can improve your sense of balance.

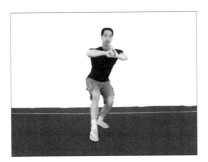 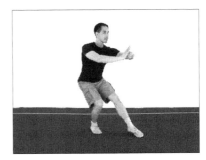

Alternate Views

Muscles Worked

Front: Abdominals, Obliques, Hip Flexors, Hip Adductors, Quads, Shin

Back: Lower Back, Gluteus Maximus, Hip Abductors, Hamstrings, Calf

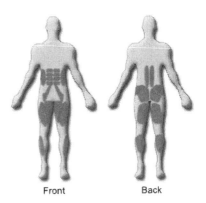

Front   Back

Basic Progressions

Cat Stance

Difficulty: ★★★☆☆

Directions

Stand with all of your weight on one leg. Keeping your back straight, but not necessarily vertical, bend that knee just past a 90-degree angle, so that the thigh is parallel to the ground. Let the foot of the free leg touch the ground lightly, making sure it does not support any of your weight.

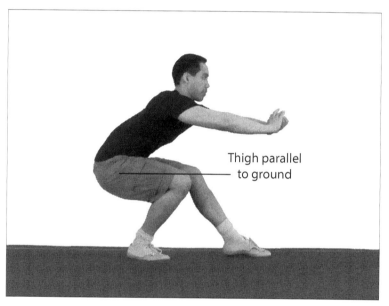

Thigh parallel to ground

Comments

This is an advanced exercise and it can be quite difficult. Try to keep the heel of the supporting foot down. While this may make the exercise a bit more difficult at first, it will provide a better overall workout.

Tips

» If you need help with balance, you can touch or hold on to something stable such as a table or wall. However, don't use it to lighten the load on your target muscles.

Basic Progressions

» The front foot should not support any of your weight. However, if you need some assistance when you are working on this exercise the first few times, you can put a little bit of your weight on the front foot. Eventually, you should wean yourself off of any support from the front leg.

» The further you can bend forward at the ankle, the easier it will be to maintain this position. If your ankles aren't flexible, you may need to hold your hands in front of you to help with your balance.

» An alternative arm position is to hold them near your body. This will make it more difficult to balance yourself and will require more leg strength. Also, the more vertical your upper body, the more difficult this exercise will be. As you get stronger, try making your upper body more vertical to improve faster.

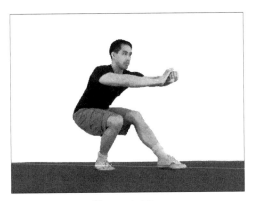

Alternate View

Muscles Worked

Front: Abdominals, Obliques, Hip Flexors, Hip Adductors, Quads, Shin

Back: Lower Back, Gluteus Maximus, Hip Abductors, Hamstrings, Calf

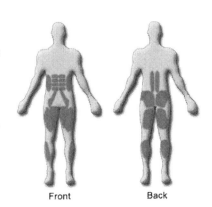

Front   Back

Pistol Squat

Difficulty: ★★★★☆

Directions

Stand with all of your weight on one leg. Lift the other leg and keep it as parallel to the ground as you can. Bend the knee of the supporting leg until that thigh is also parallel to the ground. Do not let the thigh of the bent leg rest on the calf muscle.

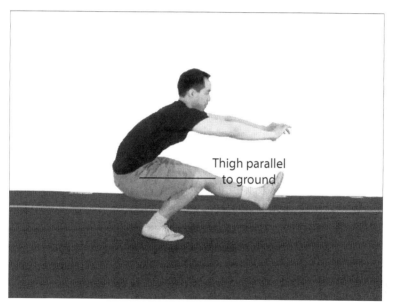

Thigh parallel to ground

Comments

This is a very difficult exercise and balance can be problematic if your ankles are not very flexible. Use a support if needed to prevent falling. As you get stronger, try to wean yourself away from using any support. Hamstring and lower back flexibility will also make it easier to hold the free leg up and parallel to the ground. Again, you may find it easier to maintain your balance by holding your hands out in front of you as a counterbalance.

Basic Progressions

Tips

» If you need help with your balance, you can touch or hold on to something stable, such as a table or wall. However, don't use it to lighten the load on your target muscles.

» If you can't go all the way down to the proper position at first, you can use your hands to hold on to a support to provide some assistance. Just make sure you use as little assistance as possible, since you want to work on your leg strength. As you get stronger, you will eventually be able to do this exercise without any assistance.

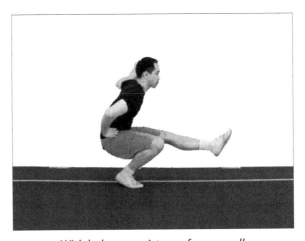

With balance assistance from a wall.

Muscles Worked

Front: Abdominals, Obliques, Hip Flexors, Hip Adductors, Quads, Shin

Back: Lower Back, Gluteus Maximus, Hip Abductors, Hamstrings, Calf

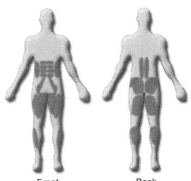

Front   Back

Basic Progressions

22

Front Leg Raises

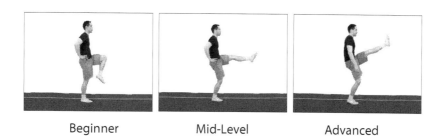

| Beginner | Mid-Level | Advanced |

The Front Leg Raise Progression focuses on core and leg strength and balance. Even though only a single leg is raised at a time, the muscles in both legs are worked, just in different ways. The muscles in the raised leg work to keep the leg raised in the proper position. The muscles in the supporting leg work together with the core muscles to provide a solid support for the muscles of the raised leg. Without a solid support, it is difficult to raise the leg to the desired position.

This progression will work on your hip flexors as well as your quads, core, and gluteus muscles. Lower back and leg flexibility will play an important role in the advanced exercises. While you can use these exercises to slowly improve your active flexibility, the advanced exercises will be more difficult until your flexibility has improved sufficiently. It may help to lightly stretch the involved muscles before doing the exercise. This will enable you to lift your leg to a higher position, working your muscles more intensely. Either way, this progression will improve your active flexibility as well as strength.

Since this progression involves standing on a single leg, balance will contribute to the difficulty of the exercise. It is important to first develop the necessary strength to perform the exercise. After that, you can work on your ability to maintain balance. If you find yourself needing some help to balance yourself during an exercise, it's okay to hold on to a table, chair, wall, or some other stable object. As you get stronger, the exercise will become easier, and you can rely less on the support. Eventually, you will be able to do the exercise without any support. At that point, you can focus on improving your sense of balance, which will work wonders on all of the muscles involved.

Equipment Needed

Floor Space
Support for balance, such as a chair or wall (optional)

Exercise Map

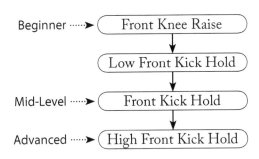

Front Knee Raise

Difficulty: ★☆☆☆☆

Directions

Stand on one leg. Bend the knee of the other leg and lift it up so that the thigh is at least parallel to the ground.

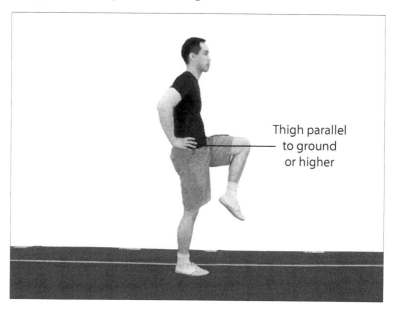

Thigh parallel to ground or higher

Basic Progressions

Comments

This exercise focuses on the hip flexors of the raised leg without worrying about the quads. Be sure to keep your supporting leg straight and make sure your upper body is as vertical as possible and in line with the supporting leg.

Tips

» You can raise your knee higher than your waist if you want. Doing so will increase the intensity of the exercise.

» Contracting your core muscles will make it easier to raise and keep your free leg up.

» Try to relax the muscles in your supporting foot so that your foot has as much contact with the floor as possible. This will make it easier for you to maintain your balance. If needed, use your hands to hold on to a support. As you get stronger, try to wean yourself off of the support.

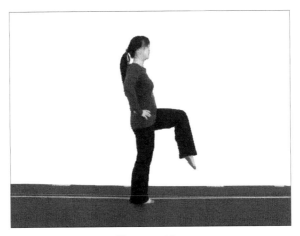

Alternate View

Muscles Worked

Front: Abdominals, Obliques, Hip Flexors, Hip Adductors, Shin

Back: Lower Back, Gluteus Maximus, Hip Abductors, Calf

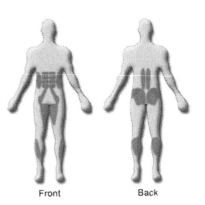

Front   Back

Low Front Kick Hold

Difficulty: ★☆☆☆☆

Directions

Stand on one leg. Raise the other leg up in front of you until it forms a 45-degree angle with your supporting leg. Be sure to keep the knee of the raised leg straight the entire time.

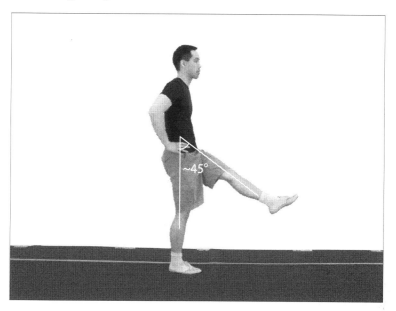

Comments

This exercise focuses on the hip flexors of the raised leg and starts working on the quads as well. Be sure to keep your supporting leg straight and make sure your upper body is as vertical as possible and in line with the supporting leg.

Tips

> » Contracting your core muscles will make it easier to raise and keep your free leg up.

> » Try to relax the muscles in your supporting foot so that your foot has as much contact with the floor as possible. This will

make it easier for you to maintain your balance. If needed, use your hands to hold on to a support. As you get stronger, try to wean yourself off of the support.

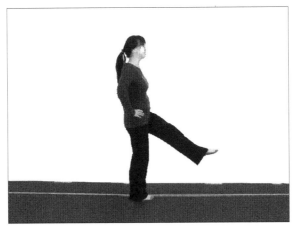

Alternate View

Muscles Worked

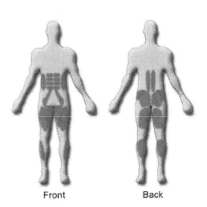

Front: Abdominals, Obliques, Hip Flexors, Hip Adductors, Quads, Shin

Back: Lower Back, Gluteus Maximus, Hip Abductors, Hamstrings, Calf

Front   Back

Front Kick Hold

Difficulty: ★★☆☆☆

Directions

Stand on one leg. Raise the other leg up in front of you until it is parallel to the ground. Be sure to keep the knee of the raised leg straight the entire time.

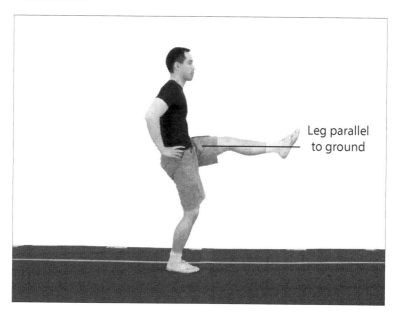

Leg parallel to ground

Comments

This exercise focuses even more intensely on the hip flexors of the raised leg. Your quads may also start to get tired earlier and cramp up. Try not to let the raised leg bend at all if you can. A tight lower back or hamstrings will make this exercise more difficult. You may feel like bending the supporting knee to relieve the tension. However, you should resist this urge and keep your supporting leg as straight as you can. Also, make sure your upper body is as vertical as possible and in line with the supporting leg. Doing so will provide more benefit in the long run.

Tips

» Contracting your core muscles will make it easier to raise and keep your free leg up.

» Try to relax the muscles in your supporting foot so that your foot has as much contact with the floor as possible. This will make it easier for you to maintain your balance. If needed, use your hands to hold on to a support. As you get stronger, try to wean yourself off of the support.

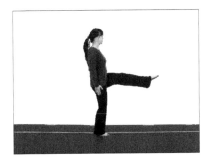 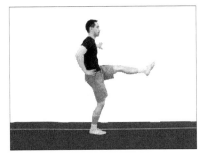

Try to keep both legs straight as in the left picture. Flexibility will make this easier to do. You can also use a support as shown on the right.

Muscles Worked

Front: Abdominals, Obliques, Hip Flexors, Hip Adductors, Quads, Shin

Back: Lower Back, Gluteus Maximus, Hip Abductors, Hamstrings, Calf

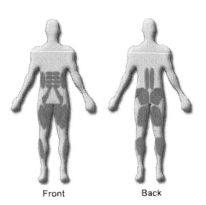

Front   Back

High Front Kick Hold

Difficulty: ★★★☆☆

Directions

Stand on one leg. Raise the other leg up in front of you until it is a foot or more above your waist. Be sure to keep the knee of the raised leg straight the entire time.

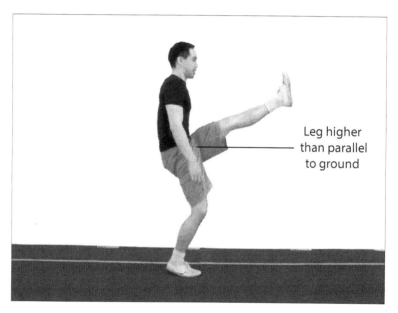

Leg higher than parallel to ground

Comments

This exercise focuses very intensely on the hip flexors and quads of the raised leg. Like the previous exercise, a tight lower back or hamstrings will make this exercise more difficult. You may feel like bending the supporting knee to relieve the tension. However, you should resist this urge and keep your supporting leg as straight as you can. Similarly, try not to let the raised leg bend at the knee. Also, make sure your upper body is as vertical as possible and in line with the supporting leg. Doing so will provide more benefit in the long run.

Tips

» Contracting your core muscles will make it easier to raise and keep your free leg up.

» Try to relax the muscles in your supporting foot so that your foot has as much contact with the floor as possible. This will make it easier for you to maintain your balance. If needed, use your hands to hold on to a support. As you get stronger, try to wean yourself off of the support.

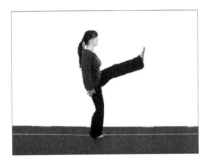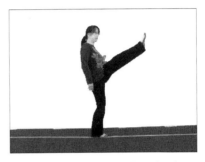

Try to keep both legs straight as in the left picture. Flexibility will make this easier to do. You can also use a support as shown on the right.

Muscles Worked

Front: Abdominals, Obliques, Hip Flexors, Hip Adductors, Quads, Shin

Back: Lower Back, Gluteus Maximus, Hip Abductors, Hamstrings, Calf

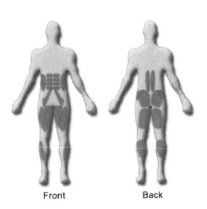

Front   Back

Basic Progressions

23

Back Leg Raises

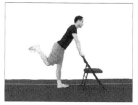 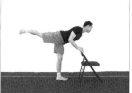 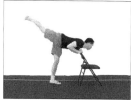

| Beginner | Mid-Level | Advanced |

The Back Leg Raise Progression focuses on core and leg strength as well as balance. Like the Front Leg Raise Progression, even though only a single leg is raised, the muscles in both legs are worked, but in different ways. The muscles in the raised leg work to keep the leg raised in the proper position. The muscles in the supporting leg work together with the core muscles to provide a solid support for the muscles of the raised leg. Without a solid support, it is difficult to raise the leg to the desired position.

This progression will work on your *gluteus* muscles as well as back core muscles. Abdominal, lower back and leg flexibility will also play an important role in the advanced exercises in this progression. While you can use these exercises to slowly improve your active flexibility, the advanced exercises will be more difficult until your flexibility has improved enough. It may help to lightly stretch the involved muscles before doing the exercise. This will enable you to lift your leg to a higher position, working your muscles more intensely. Either way, this progression will improve your active flexibility as well as strength.

Since this progression involves standing on a single leg, balance will contribute to the difficulty of the exercise. It is important to first develop the necessary strength to perform the exercise. After that, you can work on your ability to maintain balance. If you find yourself needing some help to balance yourself during an exercise, it's okay to hold on to a table, chair, wall, or some other stable object. As you get stronger, the exercise will become easier and you can rely less on the support. Eventually, you will be able to do the exercise without any support. At that point, you can focus on improving your sense of balance, which will work wonders on all of the muscles involved.

Equipment Needed

Floor Space
Support for balance, such as a chair or wall (optional)

Exercise Map

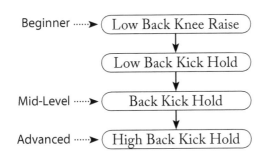

Low Back Knee Raise

Difficulty: ★☆☆☆☆

Directions

Stand on one leg. Bend the knee of the other leg and lift it back and upward until the thigh is at about a 45-degree angle to the supporting leg.

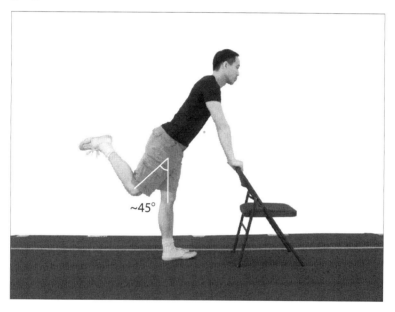

Comments

This exercise starts working on your hip extensors (e.g. gluteus muscles). Be sure to keep your hips squared toward the front. If you turn your hips out, you will be working different muscles.

Tips

» Try to relax the muscles in your supporting foot so that your foot has as much contact with the floor as possible. This will make it easier for you to maintain your balance. If needed, use your hands to hold on to a support. As you get stronger, try to wean yourself off of the support.

Basic
Progressions

Low Back Knee Raise

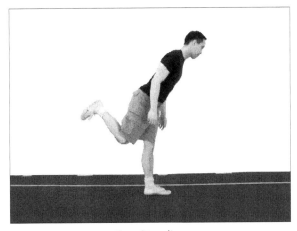

Free Standing

Muscles Worked

Front: Abdominals, Obliques, Hip Flexors, Hip Adductors, Shin

Back: Lower Back, Gluteus Maximus, Hip Abductors, Hamstrings, Calf

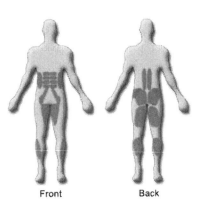

Front   Back

Low Back Kick Hold

Difficulty: ★☆☆☆☆

Directions

Stand on one leg. Keep the other leg straight and lift it back and upward until it is at about a 45-degree angle to the supporting leg.

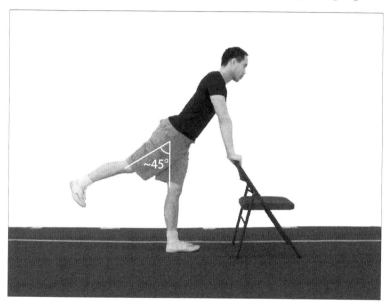

Comments

This exercise works your hip extensors, such as the *gluteus* muscles, even more because you are keeping your leg straight. Be sure to keep your hips squared toward the front. If you turn your hips out, you will be working different muscles. Try not to lean forward too much (no more than 45 degrees), since doing so will reduce the amount of work on the target muscles. Be sure to keep your supporting leg straight and vertical. You should also contract your core muscles to help maintain good posture.

Tips

» Try to relax the muscles in your supporting foot so that your foot has as much contact with the floor as possible. This will make it easier for you to maintain your balance. If needed, use your hands to hold on to a support. As you get stronger, try to wean yourself off of the support.

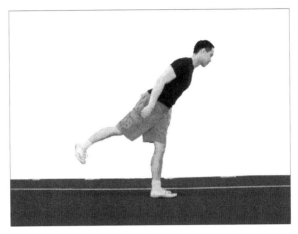

Free Standing

Muscles Worked

Front: Abdominals, Obliques, Hip Flexors, Hip Adductors, Shin

Back: Lower Back, Gluteus Maximus, Hip Abductors, Hamstrings, Calf

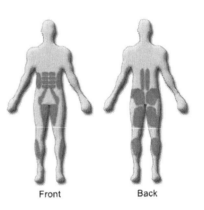

Front   Back

Basic Progressions

Back Kick Hold

Difficulty: ★★☆☆☆

Directions

Stand on one leg. Keep the other leg straight and lift it back and upward until it is parallel to the ground.

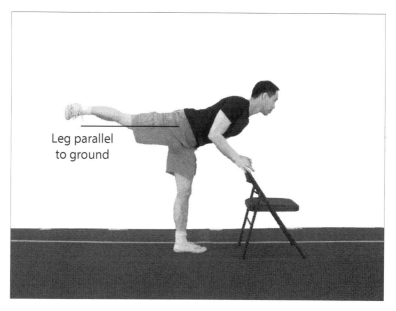

Leg parallel to ground

Comments

This exercise works on your hip extensors even more than the previous one. Again, try not to lean forward too much (not more than horizontal) so that you can engage your target muscles more. If you lean forward too far, it makes it easier for your leg muscles, but that will hinder your progress. Again, keep your hips squared to the front and the floor.

Tips

» Try to relax the muscles in your supporting foot so that your foot has as much contact with the floor as possible. This will make it easier for you to maintain your balance. If needed, use your hands to hold on to a support. As you get stronger, try to wean yourself off of the support.

Basic Progressions

» Flexibility will play a role here, especially for the supporting leg. Stretching the involved muscles a bit beforehand should make this exercise easier.

» You can turn the foot of the raised leg out to the side or keep it pointed toward the ground. You can also keep the toes dorsi-flexed (pulled up towards your head) or plantar-flexed (pointed away from your head). Even though these small variations work your muscles slightly differently, they will still provide the same general benefits.

» Remember to contract your core muscles, especially your lower back. This will help you keep your leg up.

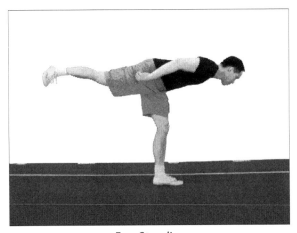

Free Standing

Muscles Worked

Front: Abdominals, Obliques, Hip Flexors, Hip Adductors, Quads, Shin

Back: Lower Back, Gluteus Maximus, Hip Abductors, Hamstrings, Calf

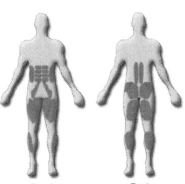

Front   Back

High Back Kick Hold

Difficulty: ★★★☆☆

Directions

Stand on one leg. Keep the other leg straight and lift it back and upward until it is a foot or higher above your waist.

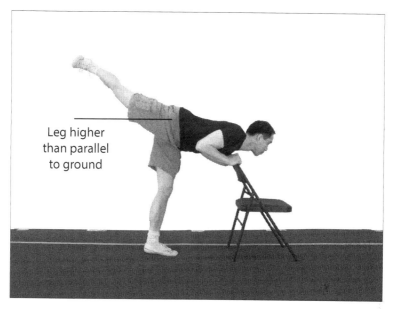

Leg higher than parallel to ground

Comments

This exercise works extensively on the hip extensors as well as your lower back muscles. Again, try not to lean down too much (not too much below horizontal) so that you can engage your target muscles more. Instead, focus on contracting your lower back and glutes as much as possible. Also, try to keep your hips squared to the front and the floor.

Tips

» Try to relax the muscles in your supporting foot so that your foot has as much contact with the floor as possible. This will make it easier for you to maintain your balance. If needed, use your hands to hold on to a support. As you get stronger, try to wean yourself off of the support.

» Flexibility in both the supporting and raised leg will play a role here. For the supporting leg, it is the flexibility of the hamstrings and to a lesser degree, the adductors. For the raised leg, it is the hip flexors and the adductors. Stretching the involved muscles a bit beforehand should make this exercise easier.

» You can turn the foot of the raised leg out to the side or keep it pointed toward the ground. You can also keep the toes dorsi-flexed (pulled up towards your head) or plantar-flexed (pointed away from your head). Even though these small variations work your muscles slightly differently, they will still provide the same general benefits.

» Remember to contract your core muscles, especially your lower back. This will help you keep your leg up.

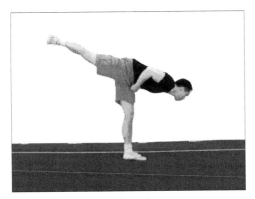

Free Standing

Muscles Worked

Front: Abdominals, Obliques, Hip Flexors, Hip Adductors, Quads, Shin

Back: Lower Back, Gluteus Maximus, Hip Abductors, Hamstrings, Calf

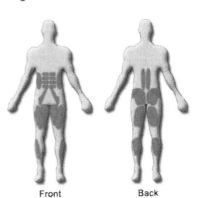

Front   Back

24

Side Leg Raises

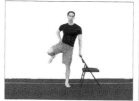 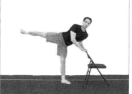 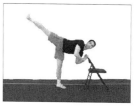

| Beginner | Mid-Level | Advanced |

The Side Leg Raise Progression focuses on core and leg strength as well as balance. Like the other Leg Raise Progressions, even though only a single leg is raised, the muscles in both legs are worked, but in different ways. The muscles in the raised leg work hard to keep the leg raised in the proper position. The muscles in the supporting leg work together with the core muscles to provide a solid support for the muscles of the raised leg. Without a solid support, it is more difficult to raise the leg to the desired position.

This progression will work on your hip abductors as well as your obliques. Leg flexibility will also play an important role in the advanced exercises. While you can use these exercises to slowly improve your active flexibility, the advanced exercises will be more difficult until your flexibility has improved enough. It may help to lightly stretch the involved muscles before doing the exercise. This will enable you to lift your leg to a higher position, working your muscles more intensely. Either way, this progression will improve your active flexibility as well as strength.

Since this progression involves standing on a single leg, balance will contribute to the difficulty of the exercise. It is important to first develop the necessary strength to perform the exercise. After that, you can work on your ability to maintain balance. If you find yourself needing some help to balance yourself during an exercise, it's okay to hold on to a table, chair, wall, or some other stable object. As you get stronger, the exercise will become easier and you can rely less on the support. Eventually, you will be able to do the exercise without any support. At that point, you can focus on improving your sense of balance, which will work wonders on all of the muscles involved.

Equipment Needed

Floor Space
Support for balance, such as a chair or wall (optional)

Exercise Map

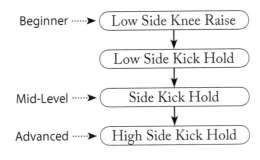

Beginner ·····▶ (Low Side Knee Raise)

(Low Side Kick Hold)

Mid-Level ·····▶ (Side Kick Hold)

Advanced ·····▶ (High Side Kick Hold)

Basic
Progressions

Low Side Knee Raise

Difficulty: ★☆☆☆☆

Directions

Stand on one leg, turning the foot out a bit to the side. Bend the knee of the other leg and raise the thigh up to the side to about a 45-degree angle to the supporting leg. Keep your upper body as vertical as possible.

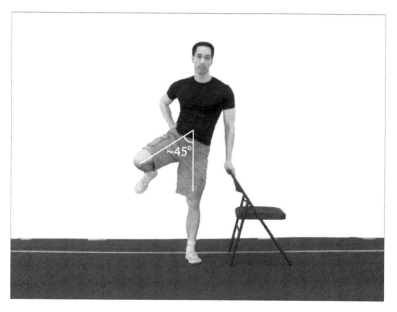

Comments

This exercise starts working on the hip abductors, which include the *gluteus medius* and *gluteus minimus* muscles. Strong hip abductors (and adductors) are important for stabilizing the hip joint. In addition, they are part of the extended core muscle group. Strengthening these muscles will help improve your ability to maintain balance.

Tips

» Try to relax the muscles in your supporting foot so that your foot has as much contact with the floor as possible. This will make it easier for you to maintain your balance. If needed, use your hands to hold on to a support. As you get stronger, try to wean yourself off of the support.

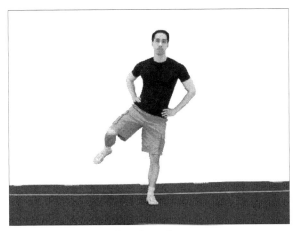

Free Standing

Muscles Worked

Front: Abdominals, Obliques, Hip Flexors, Hip Adductors, Shin

Back: Lower Back, Gluteus Maximus, Hip Abductors, Hamstrings, Calf

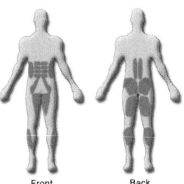

Front   Back

Low Side Kick Hold

Difficulty: ★☆☆☆☆

Directions

Stand on one leg, turning the foot out a bit to the side. Keep the other leg straight and raise the leg out to the side to about a 45-degree angle to the supporting leg. Keep your upper body as vertical as possible.

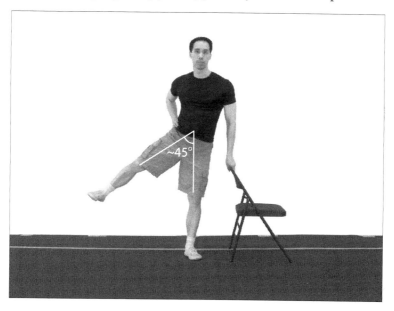

Comments

By extending your leg, this exercise works more on your hip abductors, including the *gluteus medius* and *gluteus minimus* muscles. Due to the extended leg, it will be harder to keep your upper body vertical, but do your best, since it will maximize the work your muscles will need to do.

Tips

» Try to relax the muscles in your supporting foot so that your foot has as much contact with the floor as possible. This will make it easier for you to maintain your balance. If needed, use your hands to hold on to a support. As you get stronger, try to wean yourself off of the support.

Basic Progressions

Low Side Kick Hold

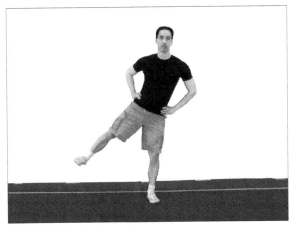

Free Standing

Muscles Worked

Front: Abdominals, Obliques, Hip Flexors, Hip Adductors, Quads, Shin

Back: Lower Back, Gluteus Maximus, Hip Abductors, Hamstrings, Calf

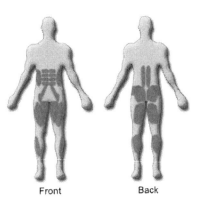

Front   Back

Side Kick Hold

Difficulty: ★★☆☆☆

Directions

Stand on one leg, turning the foot out about 90 degrees to the side. Keep the other leg straight and raise it to the side and upward until it is parallel to the ground. Try not to let your upper body bend down to the side too much (keep it above horizontal).

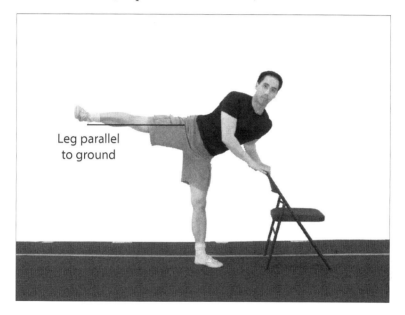

Leg parallel to ground

Comments

This exercise works intensely on your hip adductors, and to a lesser extent, your quads. Keeping your upper body up as much as you can will increase the stress on your muscles. This will also further engage your obliques. When you get tired, you may find that the knee of your raised leg will want to bend slightly. Fight this tendency and keep the leg straight and locked out. Also, do not move the raised leg toward your back even though that may feel easier. Doing so will reduce the load on the target muscles.

Tips

» Try to relax the muscles in your supporting foot so that your foot has as much contact with the floor as possible. This will make it easier for you to maintain your balance. If needed, use your hands to hold on to a support. As you get stronger, try to wean yourself off of the support.

» You can either point your toes or pull them up toward your head. Even though these variations work on the muscles in slightly different ways, both provide the same general benefits.

» Flexibility may play a role here. Stretching the involved muscles a bit beforehand should make this exercise easier.

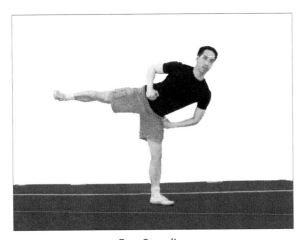

Free Standing

Muscles Worked

Front: Abdominals, Obliques, Hip Flexors, Hip Adductors, Quads, Shin

Back: Lower Back, Gluteus Maximus, Hip Abductors, Hamstrings, Calf

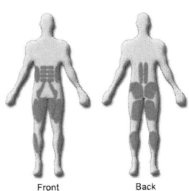

Front   Back

High Side Kick Hold

Difficulty: ★★★☆☆

Directions

Stand on one leg, turning the foot out about 90 degrees to the side. Keep the other leg straight and raise it sideways and up until it is at least a foot above your waist. Do not bend your upper body below horizontal if possible.

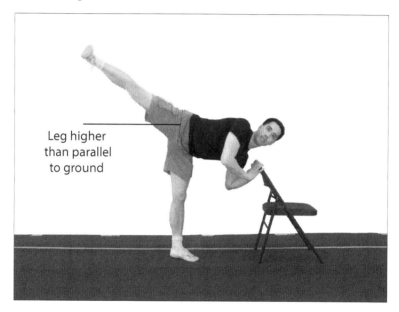

Leg higher than parallel to ground

Comments

This exercise will work very intensely on your hip adductors and also on your quads to some extent. Keeping your upper body at least horizontal or higher will increase the stress on your muscles, especially your obliques. When you get tired, you may find that the knee of your raised leg will want to bend. Fight this tendency and keep the leg straight and locked out. Also, do not move the raised leg toward your back even though that may feel easier. Doing so will reduce the load on the target muscles.

Tips

» Try to relax the muscles in your supporting foot so that your foot has as much contact with the floor as possible. This will make it easier for you to maintain your balance. If needed, use your hands to hold on to a support. As you get stronger, try to wean yourself off of the support.

» You can either point your toes or pull them up toward your head. Even though these variations work on the muscles in slightly different ways, both provide the same general benefits.

» Flexibility will definitely play a role here. Stretching the involved muscles a bit beforehand should make this exercise easier.

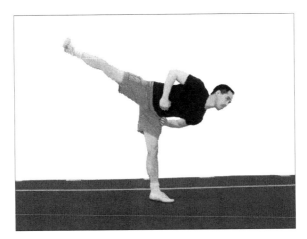

Free Standing

Muscles Worked

Front: Abdominals, Obliques, Hip Flexors, Hip Adductors, Quads, Shin

Back: Lower Back, Gluteus Maximus, Hip Abductors, Hamstrings, Calf

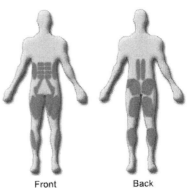

Front   Back

25

Back Lean Leg Raises

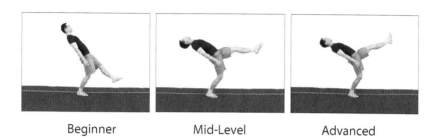

| Beginner | Mid-Level | Advanced |

The Back Lean Leg Raise Progression focuses on core and leg strength as well as balance. Leaning back with the upper body works the core muscles in a different way than the other Leg Raise Progressions. The legs also have to work differently to accommodate the change in core position. Even though only a single leg is raised, the muscles in both legs are worked, but in different ways. The muscles in the raised leg work to keep the leg raised in the proper position. The muscles in the supporting leg work with the core muscles to provide a solid support for the muscles of the raised leg. Without a solid support, it is more difficult to raise the leg to the desired position.

This progression will work on your hip flexors, quads, glutes, and front and back core muscles. Lower back and leg flexibility will play an important role in the advanced exercises. While you can use these exercises to slowly improve your active flexibility, the advanced exercises will be more difficult until your flexibility has improved enough. It may help to lightly stretch the involved muscles before doing the exercise. This will enable you to lift your leg to a higher position, working your muscles more intensely. Either way, this progression will improve your active flexibility as well as strength.

Since this progression involves standing on a single leg, balance will contribute to the difficulty of the exercise. It is important to first develop the necessary strength to perform the exercise. After that, you can work on your ability to maintain balance. If you find yourself needing some help to balance yourself during an exercise, it's okay to hold on to a table, chair, wall, or some other stable object. As you get stronger, the exercise will become easier and you can rely less on the support. Eventually, you will be able to do the exercise without any support. At that point, you can focus on improving your sense of balance, which will work wonders on all of the muscles involved in maintaining your balance for that exercise.

Equipment Needed

Floor Space
Support for balance, such as a chair or wall (optional)

Exercise Map

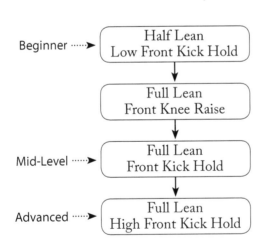

Half Lean Low Front Kick Hold

Difficulty: ★☆☆☆☆

Directions

Stand on one leg. Lean your upper body backward at the hips to about 45 degrees. At the same time, keep the other leg straight and raise it forward to a 45-degree angle from vertical.

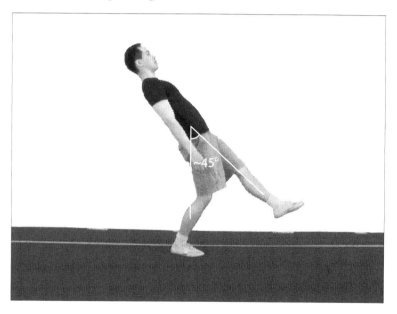

Comments

This exercise will prepare you for later exercises by strengthening your core in a reverse leveraged position.

Tips

» Focus on contracting the abs and hip flexors. Tightening up your glutes will help as well. You can let your neck tilt back a little, but it is more beneficial to keep it in a neutral position, or even tucked down toward your chest. This will help you better engage your core muscles.

Basic
Progressions

» Since you will feel this exercise intensely in your abs, make sure you remember to breathe. Take shallow breaths so that you can maintain a strong contraction in your core muscles.

» As with any single leg balance exercise, try to relax the muscles in your supporting foot so that your foot has as much contact with the floor as possible. This will make it easier for you to maintain your balance. If needed, use your hands to hold on to a support for balance. However, don't use it to lighten the load on your target muscles. As you get stronger, try to wean yourself off of the support.

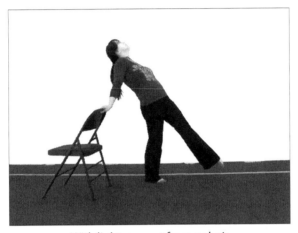

With light support from a chair.

Muscles Worked

Front: Abdominals, Obliques, Hip Flexors, Hip Adductors, Shin

Back: Lower Back, Gluteus Maximus, Hip Abductors, Calf

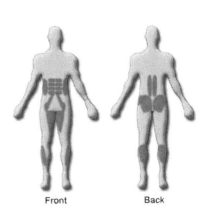

Front   Back

Full Lean Front Knee Raise

Difficulty: ★★☆☆☆

Directions

Stand on one leg. Lean your upper body backward at the hips so it is as close to parallel to the ground as you can make it. At the same time, bend the knee of the other leg and raise the thigh up in front of you until it is parallel to the ground or higher.

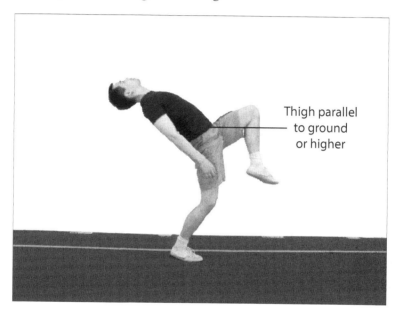

Thigh parallel to ground or higher

Comments

This exercise will further strengthen your core and hip flexors without affecting your quads too much.

Tips

» To get your knee high enough, you'll really need to focus on contracting the abs and hip flexors. Tightening up your glutes will help as well. You can let your neck tilt back a little, but it is more beneficial to keep it in a neutral position, or even tucked down toward your chest. This will help you better engage your core muscles.

» Since you will feel this exercise intensely in your abs, make sure you remember to breathe. Take shallow breaths so that you can maintain a strong contraction in your core muscles.

» As with any single leg balance exercise, try to relax the muscles in your supporting foot so that your foot has as much contact with the floor as possible. This will make it easier for you to maintain your balance. If needed, use your hands to hold on to a support for balance. However, don't use it to lighten the load on your target muscles. As you get stronger, try to wean yourself off of the support.

» An element of flexibility is needed here, especially in the abs and the hip flexors of the standing leg. Due to the weight of the upper body, this exercise will help increase the flexibility of the hip flexor. However, you will also need flexibility in the hamstrings of the raised leg in order to raise it high. It may help to stretch a bit before doing this exercise.

» If you can't lean back very far initially, don't worry. Just lean back as far as you can, holding on to a support for balance. As you get stronger and more flexible, you'll be able to lean back more and more while maintaining your raised knee at a horizontal level or higher.

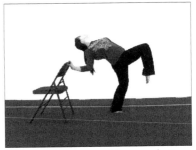

With light support from a chair.

Muscles Worked

Front: Abdominals, Obliques, Hip Flexors, Hip Adductors, Quads, Shin

Back: Lower Back, Gluteus Maximus, Hip Abductors, Hamstrings, Calf

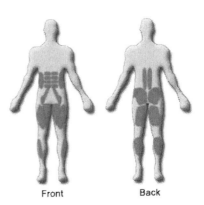

Front   Back

Full Lean Front Kick Hold

Difficulty: ★★★☆☆

Directions

Stand on one leg. Lean your upper body backward at the hips so it is as close to parallel to the ground as you can make it. At the same time, keep the other leg straight and raise it forward until it is parallel to the ground.

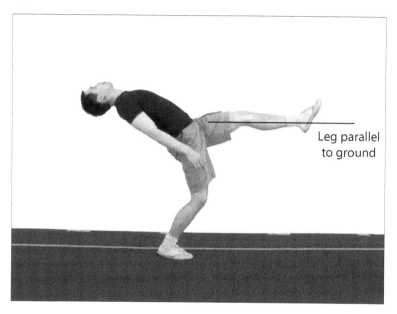

Leg parallel to ground

Basic Progressions

Comments

This exercise will work intensely on the core, especially the abs. In addition, the quads will get a workout as they struggle to keep the legs straight.

Tips

» You can let your neck tilt back a little, but it is more beneficial to keep it in a neutral position, or even tucked down toward your chest. This will help you better engage your core muscles.

» Since you will feel this exercise intensely in your abs, make sure you remember to breathe. Take shallow breaths so that you can maintain a strong contraction in your core muscles.

» As with any single leg balance exercise, try to relax the muscles in your supporting foot so that your foot has as much contact with the floor as possible. This will make it easier for you to maintain your balance. If needed, use your hands to hold on to a support for balance. However, don't use it to lighten the load on your target muscles. As you get stronger, try to wean yourself off of the support.

» You'll definitely need flexibility in the abs and hip flexors for this exercise. Again, the exercise itself will help increase the flexibility of the abs and the hip flexor of the standing leg. However, you may find that the limiting factor for the raised leg is its hamstring flexibility. It will help to stretch lightly before doing this exercise.

» If you can't lean back very far initially, don't worry. Just lean back as far as you can, holding on to a support for balance. As you get stronger and more flexible, you'll be able to lean back more and more while maintaining your raised leg at a horizontal level.

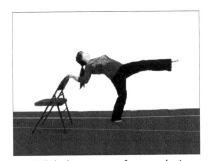

With light support from a chair.

Muscles Worked

Front: Abdominals, Obliques, Hip Flexors, Hip Adductors, Quads, Shin

Back: Lower Back, Gluteus Maximus, Hip Abductors, Hamstrings, Calf

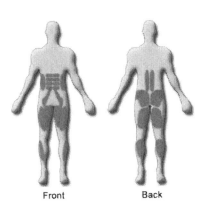

Front   Back

Full Lean High Front Kick Hold

Difficulty: ★★★★☆

Directions

Stand on one leg. Lean your upper body backward at the hips so it is as close to parallel to the ground as you can make it. At the same time, keep the other leg straight and raise it up in front of you until it is at least a foot or more above your waist.

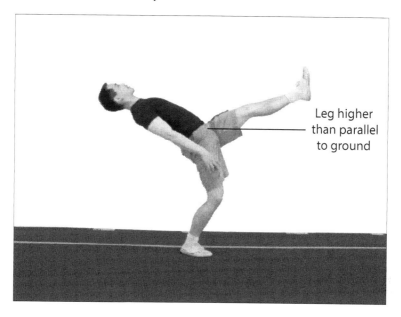

Leg higher than parallel to ground

Comments

This exercise is very difficult and will work extremely intensely on the core as well as the legs.

Tips

» You can let your neck tilt back a little, but it is more beneficial to keep it in a neutral position, or even tucked down toward your chest. This will help you better engage your core muscles.

» Since you will feel this exercise intensely in your abs, make sure you remember to breathe. Take shallow breaths so that you can maintain a strong contraction in your core muscles.

» As with any single leg balance exercise, try to relax the muscles in your supporting foot so that your foot has as much contact with the floor as possible. This will make it easier for you to maintain your balance. If needed, use your hands to hold on to a support for balance. However, don't use it to lighten the load on your target muscles. As you get stronger, try to wean yourself off of the support.

» You'll definitely need flexibility in the abs and hip flexors for this exercise. Again, the exercise itself will help increase the flexibility of the abs and the hip flexor of the standing leg. However, you may find that the limiting factor for the raised leg is its hamstring flexibility. It will help to stretch lightly before doing this exercise.

» If you can't lean back very far initially, don't worry. Just lean back as far as you can, holding on to a support for balance. As you get stronger and more flexible, you'll be able to lean back more and more while keeping your raised leg above horizontal.

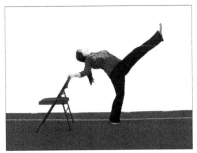

With light support from a chair.

Muscles Worked

Front: Abdominals, Obliques, Hip Flexors, Hip Adductors, Quads, Shin

Back: Lower Back, Gluteus Maximus, Hip Abductors, Hamstrings, Calf

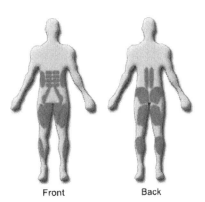

Front   Back

Advanced Progressions
&
Exercises

26

Introduction to the Advanced Progressions

This section contains the Advanced Progressions and Exercises. Depending on your level of strength and fitness, some of them can be quite tough! However, if you follow the progressions systematically and do not cheat on your form or when counting, you'll be able to make good progress. For some of the really difficult exercises, it may be hard to hold a position for a full minute (e.g. one-arm pull-up exercises). In those cases, 20 to 30 seconds or so may be sufficient to move on to the next exercise. Each person is different, so experiment and find what works best for you.

Even though you may be focused on the Advanced Progressions, you should continue to work on the exercises from the Basic Progressions. In particular, make sure you continue the progressions that work on the leg muscles. This way, you can be sure to keep your muscles as balanced as possible throughout your entire body.

Getting Stuck?

If you find your progress stalling on a particular exercise, you can try moving on to a more difficult exercise temporarily. Even though you will be doing the more difficult exercise for much shorter periods of time, the increase in difficulty may boost your strength growth. This in turn may allow you to go back to the exercise you were stalled on and master it.

Suggested Equipment

Many of the progressions in this section will require some equipment or a suitable alternative to allow you to leverage your body weight. If you don't have a particular piece of specialized equipment, try looking for something that performs the same function. For example, if you don't have a pull-up bar, you can try using the ledge of a low overhang, such as a balcony. Don't have stall bars? Try using a vertical pole, such as a solid street sign or jungle gym frame. Just make sure that whatever you are using is strong and stable enough to hold your weight. And always make sure the area around you is safe and clear before doing any of these exercises.

While the Planche and Handstand Progressions don't require any equipment, you may choose to use optional equipment to further increase the benefits you derive from those exercises. Aside from the ones described below, you can also use the push-up handles and paralletes described in the "Getting Started" chapter. If you don't have those on hand, you can even use a pair of stationary chairs or thick books as an alternative surface to work on.

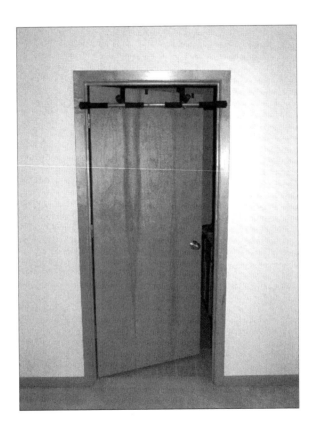

Pull-Up Bar

The pull-up bar is my second favorite piece of exercise equipment, since it is so versatile and easy to set up. You can use virtually any kind of overhanging bar as a pull-up bar. A suitable bar can usually be found at the park. If there isn't a dedicated pull-up bar there, you can just as easily use the monkey bars or the swing set. If you can't go outside, try using a door frame pull-up bar. They are easy to set up and can be taken down just as easily. You will need access to a pull-up bar or other similar support for some of the Advanced Progressions.

Rings or Suspended Handles

Rings are my favorite piece of exercise equipment. From this single piece of equipment, you can do a very large variety of exercises and develop an incredible amount of strength. Since they can (and will!) move all over the place, your muscles will work extra hard to maintain stability. I have gained more strength from working on rings than any other piece of equipment I have ever used at the gym.

Suspended handles or suspension trainers are similar to rings, except the handles are usually flat. Functionally, they are virtually identical, but

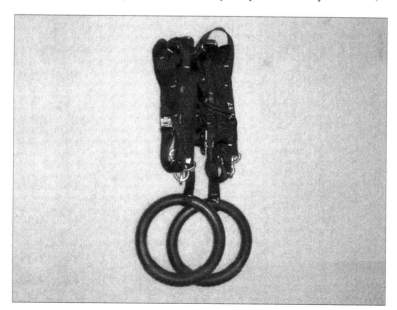

Advanced
Progressions

it is more comfortable to do certain moves on rings because they are round. Personally, I prefer the rings because it is easier to hold them in different ways to provide various levels of assistance when needed.

Finding a place to set up your exercise rings can be a challenge. You will need to hang them high enough that the rings are at least at waist level. You can mount them to supports in the ceiling, or you can hang them from an overhead bar, such as a pull-up bar, swing set at the park, or even a strong tree branch.

Try to make the straps as long as possible in order to maximize the instability effect of the rings. The shorter the straps, the easier the rings will be to use. This means less of a workout for your muscles.

Hanging the rings shoulder-width apart will maximize usability and the instability effect. If you hang them closer than that, it will make the rings easier to use. Go wider and you will find yourself constantly trying to pull the rings in. This will make it really hard to even get started with any of the exercises. Personally, I set up my rings 50 cm apart because that is how they are set up for competitive gymnastics.

If you have trouble finding a place to hang them, you can always hang them from the neutral grip handles of a doorway pull-up bar. These grips stick out just enough that the rings can clear the door frame

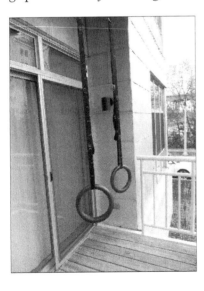
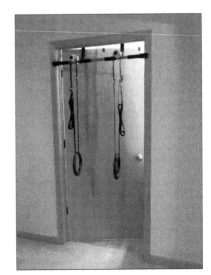

during an exercise. The downside is that the straps will be on the short side, which decreases their instability. However, it will still be enough for you to develop massive strength.

Stall Bars / Vertical Pole

Stall bars are a set of horizontally-mounted bars. They are great for working the Flag Progression. I don't expect many people to have access to these as they are usually found in gymnastics gyms. However, I have included them here for completeness. You can just as easily use a strong vertical pole such as the vertical support of an exercise station

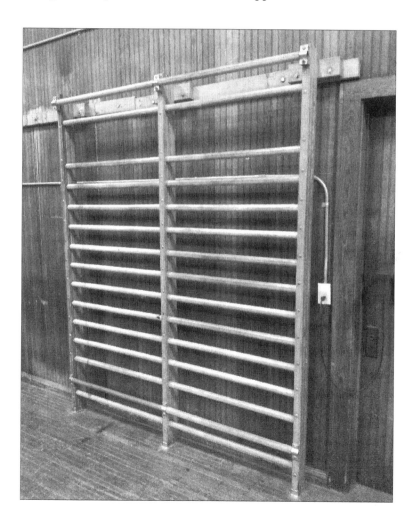

at the park. Alternatively, you can create a set up similar to stall bars by using the adjustable bars in a squat cage. You can see an example of the squat cage setup in the Flag Progression chapter. Personally, I use a door frame pull-up bar and a stable chair right below it to simulate the stall bars. If you choose to use the same setup, make sure the bar and chair don't move, tip, or slide under load.

Grip Variations

There are several grips that you can use when exercising on a pull-up bar or exercise rings. Using different grips will target your muscles slightly differently. Find the one that feels the most comfortable to you or switch them up to provide variety.

Overhand Grip

To use an overhand grip, place the palm of your hand on the bar so that it faces away from you. This pronates your wrist, which is the same direction you would rotate your wrist when placing your palm flat on the top of a table. This grip tends to target the lats a bit more than the biceps in pull-up type movements.

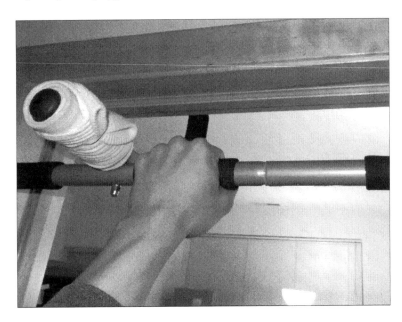

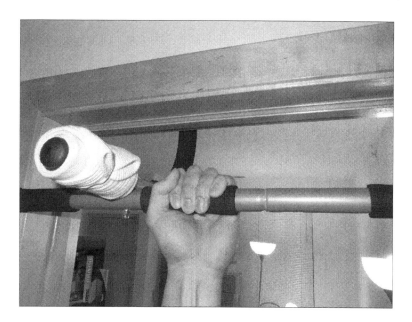

Underhand Grip

To use an underhand grip, place the palm of your hand on the bar so that it faces toward you. This supinates your wrist, which is how you would turn your wrist when placing your hand on a table with your palm facing up. This grip tends to target the biceps a bit more than the lats in pull-up type movements.

Mixed Grip

The mixed grip is a combination of the above two grips. One hand uses the overhand grip while the other hand uses the underhand grip. It is a good idea to switch up the hands throughout your workout so that you train both sides of your body evenly.

Neutral Grip

When using the neutral grip, the palms of your hands are facing each other. Generally, you will only be able to use this grip on rings, or pull-up bars that have handles designed for it. As the name suggests, this grip doesn't favor one set of muscles over another as the overhand and underhand grips do.

Advanced
Progressions

False Grip

The false grip is commonly used when combining pushing and pulling in a single movement. Using a false grip makes it easier to transition from the pulling phase to the pushing phase because the base of your palm is already on top of the support, as opposed to the overhand, underhand, and neutral grips, where it is below the support.

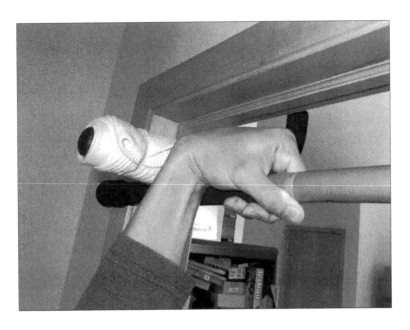

To use the false grip on a bar, place the base of your hand on top of the bar. You should feel the bar tucked into the bend of your wrist. Next, wrap your fingers around the bar as best as you can. When you put your full weight on this grip, make sure you grip the bar tightly enough so that your palm does not slip away from the top of the bar. The false grip will feel uncomfortable the first few times you use it, but you will get used to it after a while.

Using a false grip on the rings is similar to the bar. Put your hand through the ring, then place the base of your palm on top of the bottom portion of the ring. You should feel the ring tucked into where your wrist meets the base of your hand. Next, wrap your fingers around the ring. This should be a bit easier than on the bar due to the curved nature of the ring. That's it! When you put your full weight on the rings, make sure to hold on tightly so that your palm doesn't slip down below the ring. As with the bar, it will feel awkward at first, but you will get used to it before long.

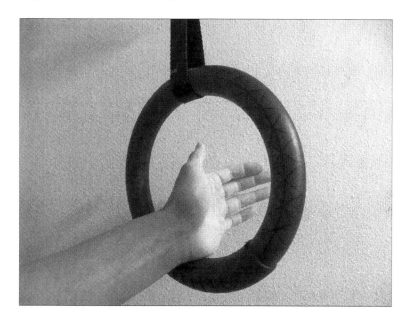

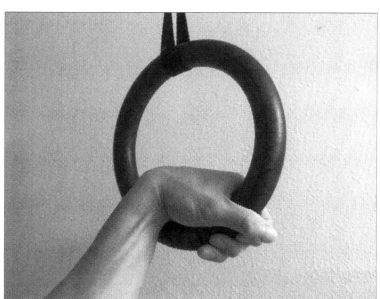

27

Planches

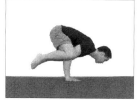 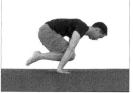 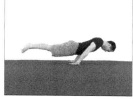

Beginner   Mid-Level   Advanced

The Planche Progression is quite advanced and requires both strength and balance. At the end of this progression, you will be able to hold yourself in a gravity-defying position where your body is parallel to the ground, like the top of a push-up position, but with your feet off the ground. Only your hands will be touching the ground! This requires a tremendous amount of strength throughout the entire body and training for it is an excellent full-body exercise.

Equipment Needed

Floor Space

These exercises are commonly performed on the ground, but they can also be done on dumbbells, paralletes, push-up handles, rings, etc. In general, flat surfaces are harder to work on than stable handles or bar-like supports because the latter provides more leverage, which you can use to help maintain your balance. In addition, the slight elevation from using these supports will make it easier to raise your feet off the floor in the later exercises. However, do not let the extra height advantage make you lazy. Make sure you maintain the proper body position for each exercise, or you will not be able to progress to the more difficult ones. There are no shortcuts here. On the other hand, working on the rings will increase difficulty significantly. It is best to be proficient performing an exercise on the ground before moving up to the unstable rings.

General Notes

There are a few keys to these exercises that will make them a bit easier. The first key is making sure you protract your shoulders as much as possible. Protracting your shoulders means pulling your shoulder blades forward and to the side. An easy way to think about it is squeezing your shoulders together in the front. This action stabilizes your upper body and shoulder position so that there is a stable support from which to extend the rest of your torso and legs.

Another key is keeping your arms straight with your elbow pits facing forward. At first, you will feel like bending your elbows because it makes the exercises easier. However, this is improper form and will not build as much strength. On the other hand, turning your elbow pits forward will help increase the amount of strength you can generate by further stabilizing your shoulders. Depending on your strength profile, this may or may not feel natural to you. I had this problem until I found out squeezing my upper arms down and together turned my elbows in the correct direction. Once I figured this out, I was able to make progress much faster.

Finally, you need to lean forward as much as possible. In order to reach the balance point for the full planche, you essentially need to put your hips over your hands. This requires a lot of shoulder strength in addition to pressing and core strength. We will go over some supplemental exercises that you can add to your routine if you are having trouble progressing from one exercise to a more difficult one.

Since these exercises involve an element of balance, there is always a possibility that you will fall out of the position. Be sure to do these exercises in an area clear of objects that you may hit if you fall. Pay special attention to the area near your head. It will be wise to work out with a soft surface that you can land on, such as towel or cushion, until you become comfortable with each exercise.

Advanced Progressions

Supplemental Exercises

If you find yourself hitting a plateau and having trouble advancing to a more difficult exercise, try adding one or both of the following supplemental exercises. They will help build additional strength and range of motion, which can help bridge the gap to the next exercise.

Front Planche Lean

This exercise simulates the feeling of going into a planche position, except your feet stay on the ground. It will help you develop the shoulder strength necessary to lean forward for other positions in the Planche Progression.

Start in a front plank position and protract your shoulders. Think about squeezing them together in the front so your upper back arches, like a cat's. Next, slowly lean forward at the shoulders while keeping your upper body and hips parallel to the ground. Keep leaning forward until the point at which you feel like you will fall out of the position. This is the maximum amount you are able to lean forward at your current strength level. Hold this position for as long as you can, up to one minute. As you get stronger, try to lean forward farther than before. This will help you develop the strength necessary to advance through these exercises.

Pseudo-Planche Push-Ups

While these may look similar to regular push-ups, they are much harder to do and provide results significantly faster. Start out in a push-up position, then lean forward as you would in a front planche lean. To perform the push-up, bend your elbows and lower your body close to the ground while keeping your shoulders ahead of your hands, just as they were at the top of the push-up. You will feel the urge to shift your body backward to reduce the load on your shoulders. However, resist this urge and keep your shoulders ahead of your hands. This will help build strength in your shoulders.

Advanced
Progressions

When you push up, make sure to keep leaning forward so that you end up with the same amount of forward lean as when you started. Your body will want to shift back as you push up, since doing so reduces the load on your muscles. Resist this by thinking about pushing down and back toward your hips during the entire upward movement. This will help you maintain the forward lean throughout the push-up. Also, be sure to keep your core tight and back straight throughout the entire exercise. Do not let your torso sag down.

As you get stronger, you can try leaning farther forward to increase difficulty. You can also raise your feet up on a chair or some other platform. This will increase the load on your muscles even more. Eventually, you'll find your feet barely touching the floor as you push up to the top of each repetition.

Exercise Map

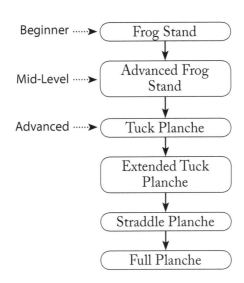

Frog Stand

Difficulty: ★✭☆☆☆

Directions

Place your hands shoulder-width apart on the ground in front of you. Bend your elbows, then place your knees by your elbows. Lean forward and transfer your weight to your hands until your feet leave the ground. Your thighs will rest on the backs of your elbows. Hold your knees up on the outsides of your elbows.

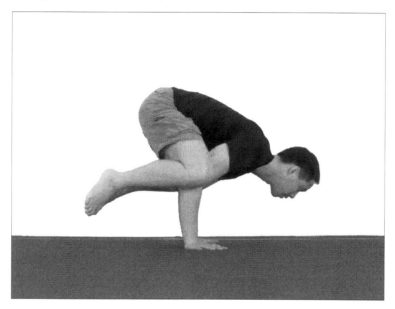

Comments

This first exercise uses a bent arm for support to make it easier. The goal here is to get used to putting all of your weight on your hands and keeping your feet off the ground without having to worry about back strength. Even though you can rest your thighs on your elbows, minimize your dependence on them by pressing down and protracting your shoulders. Doing so will better prepare you for the later exercises.

Tips

> » There are several hand positions that you can use. If your fingers are facing forward, it will be easier to balance yourself, since you

can press down with your fingers to help. As you progress to the more difficult exercises, you will need to lean forward more and more. Depending on your wrist flexibility, you may find that it is more comfortable to turn your hands out to the sides, or even toward the back. Try different hand positions and see what works for you.

» If you use rings or bar-type supports, you will need to turn your hands out to the side or backward. The most difficult hand position is where your fingers are facing backward because you will not be able to use them to help with balance. That job will fall to your shoulders. It generally takes longer to make progress with this hand position, but the control you develop will come in handy when you work the advanced exercises on the rings.

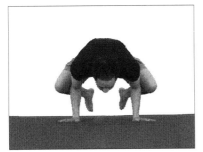

Front View

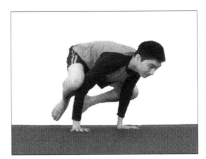

Oblique View

Muscles Worked

Front: Pectorals, Front Deltoids, Abdominals, Serratus

Back: Rear Deltoids, Rotator Cuff, Triceps, Trapezius, Lats, Rhomboids, Lower Back

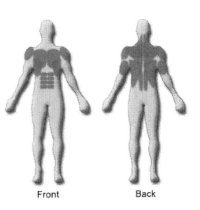

Front   Back

Advanced Frog Stand

Difficulty: ★★⯨☆☆

Directions

Place your hands shoulder-width apart on the ground in front of you. Keep your elbows straight and place your knees on the backs of your arms, just above your elbows. Lean forward and transfer your weight to your hands until your feet leave the ground.

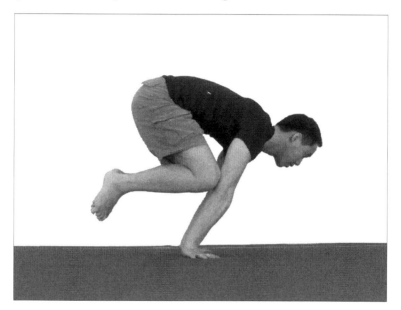

Comments

This is the first exercise to use a straight arm support and introduce reverse leverage. Even though this exercise may look similar to the Frog Stand, the straight arm requirement makes it more difficult.

Tips

» This position requires you to lean forward more, which may take a while to get used to. It is okay if you find yourself falling out of it in the beginning. Just make sure the area around you is free of objects that you might fall on. Eventually, you will develop the strength and balance necessary to hold the position.

Advanced Progressions

Advanced Frog Stand

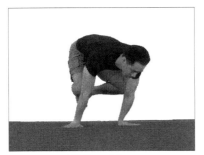

Oblique View

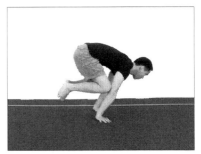

Alternate Side View

Muscles Worked

Front: Pectorals, Front Deltoids, Biceps, Wrist Flexors, Abdominals, Obliques, Serratus, Hip Flexors

Back: Rear Deltoids, Rotator Cuff, Triceps, Trapezius, Lats, Rhomboids, Lower Back, Hamstrings

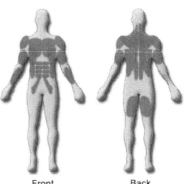

Front   Back

Tuck Planche

Difficulty: ★★★☆☆

Directions

Place your hands shoulder-width apart on the ground in front of you. Keep your arms straight and lift your hips until your back is parallel to the ground or slightly higher. Lean forward and transfer your weight to your hands until your feet leave the ground. You may need to pull your knees up tightly to your chest so that your feet can clear the ground. Do not rest your knees or legs against your arms. You can keep your back rounded.

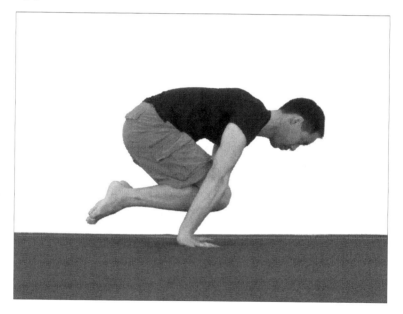

Comments

If you are working on elevated supports or rings, you can also work on tuck planche push-ups. To do these, first start in a tuck planche. Bend your elbows to dip down, then press up and forward before your feet touch the ground. You will need to focus on balance here because the balance point shifts as you go up and down. Remember to push down and back toward your hips in order to maintain the necessary forward lean.

Tips

» The key here is to lean forward enough while keeping your hips up. You will need to contract your abs and hip flexors tightly to help keep your feet off the ground. At the same time, you will also need to protract the shoulders and engage the upper back muscles to maintain the necessary clearance for your feet.

» If you can't keep your fingers facing forward, try rotating them out to the side a bit to reduce the pressure on your wrists.

» From this exercise onward, if you are having difficulty advancing because you can't lean forward enough, try doing some Front Planche Leans and Pseudo-Planche Push-Ups. They will help build shoulder strength so you can lean forward more. See the instructions earlier in this chapter.

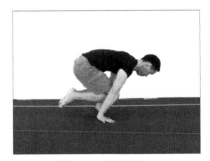

Alternate Side View

Muscles Worked

Front: Pectorals, Front Deltoids, Biceps, Wrist Flexors, Abdominals, Obliques, Serratus, Hip Flexors

Back: Rear Deltoids, Rotator Cuff, Triceps, Trapezius, Lats, Rhomboids, Lower Back, Hamstrings

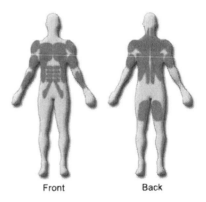

Front   Back

Extended Tuck Planche

Difficulty: ★★★★☆

Directions

Place your hands shoulder-width apart on the ground in front of you. Keep your arms straight and lift your hips until your back is straight and parallel to the ground or slightly higher. Lean forward and transfer your weight to your hands until your feet leave the ground. Remember to keep your back straight, not rounded.

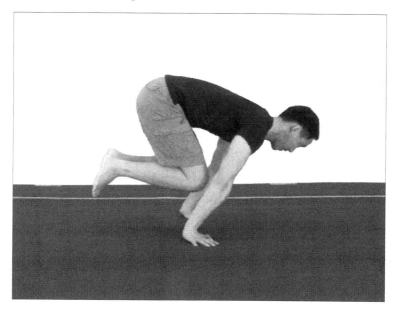

Comments

Even though the difference between this exercise and the regular Tuck Planche appears minor (rounded vs. straight back), the increase in difficulty is significant. Extending the back so that it is straight increases reverse leverage significantly. It will require even more of a forward lean and a lot more core strength. If you are working on elevated supports or rings, you can also work on Extended Tuck Planche Push-Ups.

Tips

» If you can't lean far enough forward, work on Forward Planche Leans and Pseudo-Planche Push-Ups.

Advanced Progressions

» If you can't keep your fingers facing forward, try rotating them out to the side a bit to reduce the pressure on your wrists.

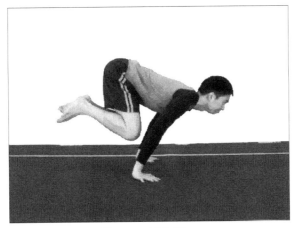

Alternate Side View

Muscles Worked

Front: Pectorals, Front Deltoids, Biceps, Wrist Flexors, Abdominals, Obliques, Serratus, Hip Flexors

Back: Rear Deltoids, Rotator Cuff, Triceps, Trapezius, Lats, Rhomboids, Lower Back, Gluteus Maximus, Hamstrings

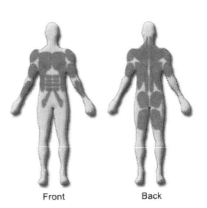

Front   Back

Advanced
Progressions

Straddle Planche

Difficulty: ★★★★★

Directions

Place your hands shoulder-width apart on the ground in front of you. Keep your arms straight and lift your hips until your back is straight and parallel to the ground or slightly higher. Lean forward and transfer your weight to your hands until your feet leave the ground. Extend your legs straight and out to the sides in a straddle position. Remember to keep your back straight, not rounded.

Alternatively, you can start in a standing straddle position and lean forward on to your hands until your feet leave the ground and your lower body is extended in the proper position.

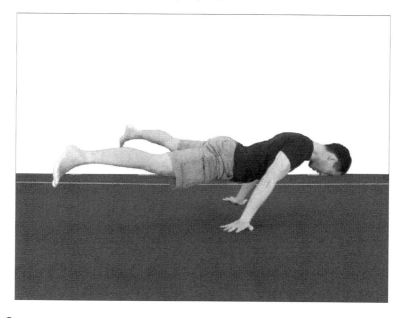

Comments

The straddle position allows you to start working on straight leg planche work without requiring the strength for a fully extended, legs-together planche.

Tips

»   It may be difficult to straddle your legs in the prone position at first. If that is the case, and you have access to a pull-up bar or other suitable support to hang from, work on Straddle Back Levers.

»   Be sure to keep your arms straight. Even a slight bend will make it feel much easier, but this incorrect form will prevent you from moving on to the full planche. However, working on Straddle Planche Push-Ups is a great way to build up additional strength.

»   If you can't keep your fingers facing forward, try rotating them out to the side a bit to reduce the pressure on your wrists.

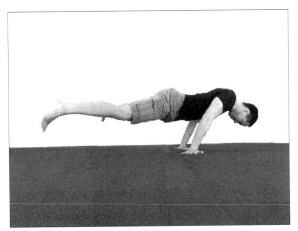

Alternate Side View

Muscles Worked

Front: Pectorals, Front Deltoids, Biceps, Wrist Flexors, Abdominals, Obliques, Serratus, Hip Flexors, Hip Adductors, Quads

Back: Rear Deltoids, Rotator Cuff, Triceps, Trapezius, Lats, Rhomboids, Lower Back, Gluteus Maximus, Hip Abductors, Hamstrings

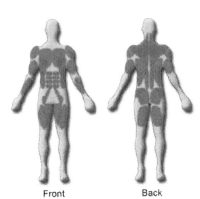

Front   Back

Advanced Progressions

Full Planche

Difficulty: ★★★★★ +

Directions

Place your hands shoulder-width apart on the ground in front of you. Keep your arms straight and lift your hips until your back is straight and parallel to the ground or slightly higher. Lean forward and transfer your weight to your hands until your feet leave the ground. Keeping your legs together, extend your legs straight back. Remember to keep your back straight, not rounded.

Alternatively, you can start at the bottom of a Planche Push-Up and then push up into the Full Planche. However, this requires you to already be able to do a Full Planche Push-Up.

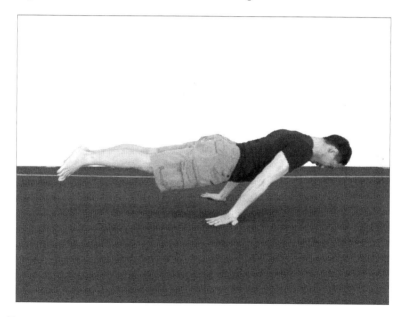

Comments

This exercise is intensely difficult and requires strength in your entire body. The ability to do a Full Back Lever is a prerequisite, or you will have difficulty keeping your body fully extended in the air.

Advanced
Progressions

Tips

» Having trouble with the Full Planche? Do Straddle Planche Push-Ups to help build up additional strength.

» If you can't keep your fingers facing forward, try rotating them out to the side a bit to reduce the pressure on your wrists.

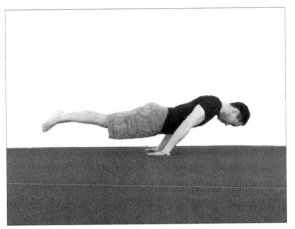

Alternate Side View

Muscles Worked

Front: Pectorals, Front Deltoids, Biceps, Wrist Flexors, Abdominals, Obliques, Serratus, Hip Flexors, Hip Adductors, Quads

Back: Rear Deltoids, Rotator Cuff, Triceps, Trapezius, Lats, Rhomboids, Lower Back, Gluteus Maximus, Hip Abductors, Hamstrings

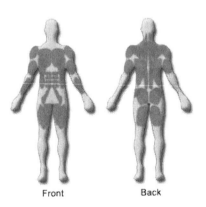

Front   Back

Advanced Progressions

28

Handstands

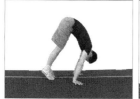 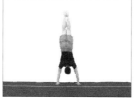 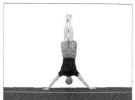

Beginner   Mid-Level   Advanced

The Handstand Progression is an excellent way to develop strong arms and shoulders while increasing body awareness at the same time. Being upside down may be foreign to you, but with time, it can become second nature. As you learn to become comfortable being upside down, you will learn a lot of things about controlling your body that you take for granted when upright. This increased awareness will lead to better core strength, strength usage, and overall balance.

Equipment Needed

A wall and floor space next to it that is clear of obstacles

While you can do most of these exercises without a wall or other suitable support, it is much easier with one. It allows you to focus on building strength without worrying about losing your balance and falling over. In addition, support from the wall will make the exercises a little easier when you get tired. When you have developed enough strength, you can start moving your handstand work away from the wall. With the necessary strength, it will be much easier for you to work on the balance component.

General Notes

All of the exercises in this progression, except the ones in the Arms Forward branch, which move away from the wall, can be done either with your back or front to the wall. It is generally easier to get into position with your back to the wall. The downside is that it is easy to develop poor form and bad habits, such as arching your back. Doing handstand work with your front facing the wall encourages better form and body lines. At first, it may be a little tricky learning how to get up onto and down off the wall. However, with some practice, it will become much easier. The benefits of training with your front facing the wall are well worth the extra effort. If you are new to handstands, you may want to start training with your back facing the wall. Later, when you feel comfortable, you can switch to the other way.

Getting into a handstand with your back facing the wall is fairly straightforward. Place your hands on the ground near the wall and kick your legs up gently toward the wall. Make sure to let your hips ride up with the kick so that your back doesn't arch too much. The goal is to get your feet, knees, hips, shoulders, and hands all stacked vertically on top of each other. If you don't make it all the way up at first, try again and kick a little harder and lead more with the hips. However, try not to kick too hard because you will overshoot the handstand position. Besides possibly hurting yourself and damaging the wall, you won't learn where the balance point is for a handstand.

There are a few ways to get up into a handstand facing the wall. One way is to stand with your back to the wall and place your hands on the ground. Then, walk your feet up the wall as you walk your hands in toward the wall until you reach the desired handstand position. Another way is to stand sideways in front of the wall next to where you want to do the handstand. Make a quarter-turn with your body as you bring your hands down into position and kick up into a handstand. This is similar to doing a quarter pirouette into a handstand.

Once you get up into a handstand facing the wall, you will need to be able to come down safely. You should always check to make sure you have enough clear space around you before you go into a handstand. If you have enough space, you can lower your body down slowly so your head comes near the ground. Next, tuck your head toward your chest and continue lowering your body down to the floor while pushing off the wall with your feet. This will make you roll forward on the ground. Another way is to turn away from the wall so that you can bring your feet down. This is essentially pirouetting away from the wall. All of this may seem confusing at first, but once you try it a few times, it will be easier to understand.

Exercise Map

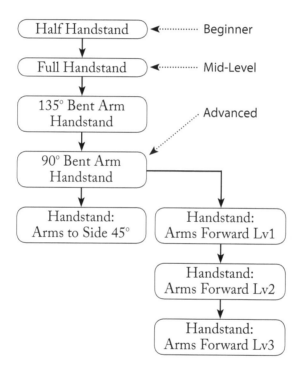

Advanced
Progressions

Half Handstand

Difficulty: ★☆☆☆☆

Directions

Place your hands on the ground near a wall. Keeping your legs straight and your feet on the ground, lean forward against the wall so that you feel your weight on your hands. If you are strong enough, you can also do this exercise without a wall.

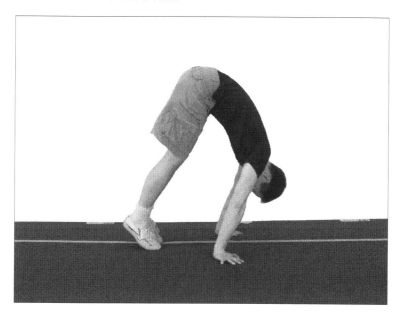

Comments

The goal here is to put as much of your weight on your hands as you can. This will get you used to having weight on your hands, and being upside down. Try to get your hands as close as possible to the wall, but they do not need to be touching it.

Tips

» If you want, you can go up on your toes to load more of your weight onto your hands.

Advanced Progressions

Half Handstand

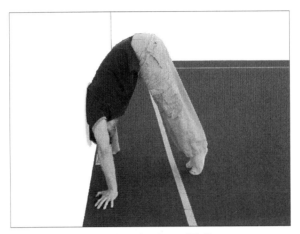

Leaning Against a Wall

Muscles Worked

Front: Pectorals, Front Deltoids, Wrist Flexors, Abdominals, Obliques, Serratus

Back: Rear Deltoids, Rotator Cuff, Triceps, Trapezius, Lats, Rhomboids, Lower Back

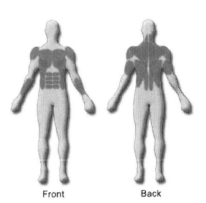

Front   Back

Full Handstand

Difficulty: ★☆☆☆☆

Directions

Place your hands on the ground near a wall. Kick or press up into a handstand against the wall.

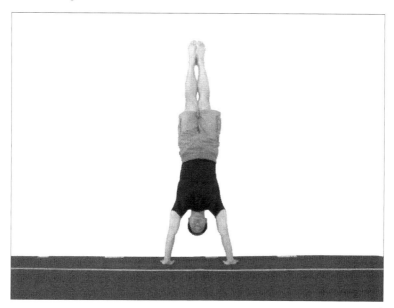

Comments

This exercise will help you get used to having your entire weight on your hands. Try to eliminate any arching in your back by starting with your hands as close to the wall as possible.

Tips

  » Keep your body tight and vertical at all times by maintaining a slight hollow in your chest and squeezing your legs together. Just as importantly, make sure to keep your shoulders shrugged toward your ears. This will help extend your body and make it easier to maintain your balance. Your core and legs should be kept straight and tight the entire time so that the support forces generated by your hands can be transmitted up to the rest of your body.

Advanced Progressions

» At first, you can look down at the ground between your hands. However, as you become more comfortable with the handstand position, you should try looking back across the floor where you were standing before going into the handstand. This neutral head position will align your body better and make it easier to balance yourself. It will also improve your overall handstand shape.

Variations

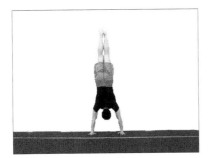

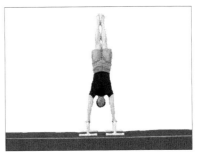

Facing a Wall   *On Paralletes*

Muscles Worked

Front: Pectorals, Front Deltoids, Wrist Flexors, Abdominals, Obliques, Serratus, Hip Flexors, Hip Adductors, Quads

Back: Rear Deltoids, Rotator Cuff, Triceps, Wrist Extensors, Trapezius, Lats, Rhomboids, Lower Back, Gluteus Maximus, Hip Abductors, Hamstrings

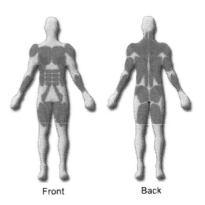

Front   Back

135° Bent Arm Handstand

Difficulty: ★★☆☆☆

Directions

Place your hands on the ground near a wall. Kick or press up into a handstand against the wall. Bend your elbows so that they form a 135-degree angle.

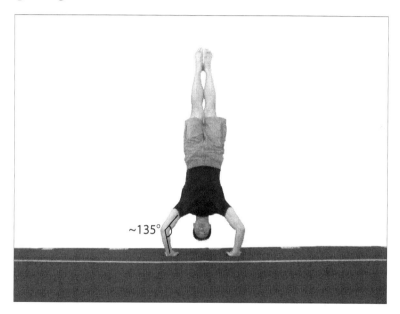

Comments

Holding your elbows bent makes this exercise more difficult. Make sure you keep your elbows squeezed together so they are as parallel to each other as you can make them. Do not let them flare out to the sides. Though that may feel easier, it will slow down your progress to more advanced exercises.

Tips

> » If you are doing this exercise with your back facing the wall, you will need to place your hands a few inches from the wall when you start. This will give you room to lower your body down without flaring your elbows out.

» If you are doing this exercise with your front facing the wall, you will need to lower your body so that your shoulders are a bit in front of your hands. This way, you can keep your elbows parallel to each other instead of flared out to the sides. This is the position you will need to achieve in order to maintain your balance when you are doing the freestanding version of this exercise (without a wall or similar support).

» You can do this exercise with your fingers facing forward or out to the sides. The different hand positions will target your muscles in different ways. Turning them out to the sides will mimic the hand position used when doing handstands on parallettes or rings. It will also make it harder for your elbows to flare out.

Variations

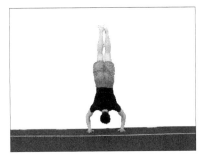

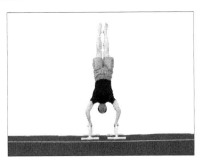

Facing a Wall   *On Parallettes*

Muscles Worked

Front: Pectorals, Front Deltoids, Wrist Flexors, Abdominals, Obliques, Serratus, Hip Flexors, Hip Adductors, Quads

Back: Rear Deltoids, Rotator Cuff, Triceps, Wrist Extensors, Trapezius, Lats, Rhomboids, Lower Back, Gluteus Maximus, Hip Abductors, Hamstrings

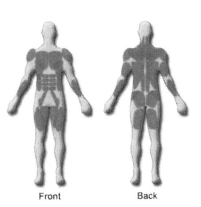

Front   Back

Advanced Progressions

90° Bent Arm Handstand

Difficulty: ★★✭☆☆

Directions

Place your hands on the ground near a wall. Kick or press up into a handstand against the wall. Bend your elbows so that they form a 90-degree angle. Your head should be just off the ground.

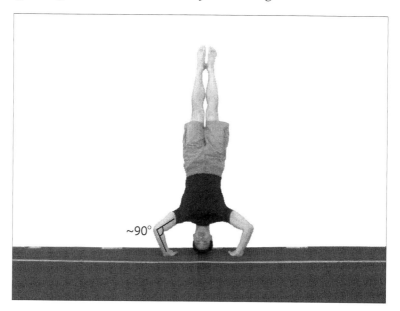

Comments

Holding your elbows bent makes this exercise more difficult. Make sure you keep your elbows squeezed together so they are as parallel to each other as you can make them. Do not let them flare out to the sides. Though that may feel easier, it will slow down your progress to more advanced exercises.

Tips

» If you are doing this exercise with your back facing the wall, you will need to place your hands a few inches from the wall when you start. This will give you room to lower your body without flaring your elbows out.

Advanced Progressions

» If you are doing this exercise with your front facing the wall, you will need to lower your body so that your shoulders are a bit in front of your hands. This way, you can keep your elbows parallel to each other instead of flared out to the sides. This is the position you will need to achieve in order to maintain your balance when you are doing the freestanding version of this exercise (without a wall or similar support).

» You can do this exercise with your fingers facing forward or out to the sides. The different hand positions will target your muscles in different ways. Turning them out to the sides will mimic the hand position used when doing handstands on paralletes or rings. It will also make it harder for your elbows to flare out.

Variations

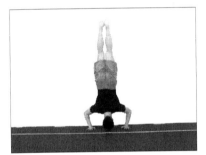

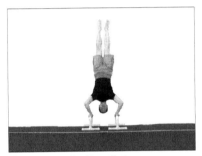

Facing a Wall   *On Paralletes*

Muscles Worked

Front: Pectorals, Front Deltoids, Wrist Flexors, Abdominals, Obliques, Serratus, Hip Flexors, Hip Adductors, Quads

Back: Rear Deltoids, Rotator Cuff, Triceps, Wrist Extensors, Trapezius, Lats, Rhomboids, Lower Back, Gluteus Maximus, Hip Abductors, Hamstrings

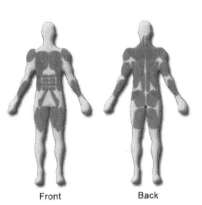

Front   Back

Handstand: Arms to Side 45°

Difficulty: ★★★☆☆

Directions

Place your hands on the ground near a wall about two shoulder-widths apart. Kick or press up into a handstand against the wall.

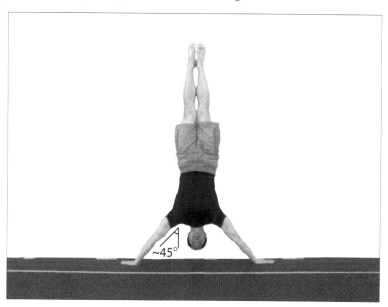

Comments

This exercise works your shoulders in a different way than the previous exercises. Due to the position of the straight arms, you will also be working your biceps. Your core and legs should be kept straight and tight the entire time so that the support forces generated by your hands can be transmitted up to the rest of your body.

Tips

» You may find it helpful to turn your hands out to the sides. Besides being more comfortable, you may get more traction this way.

» At first, you can look down at the ground between your hands. However, as you become more comfortable with the handstand position, you should try looking back across the floor where you were standing before going into the handstand. This neutral head position will align your body better and make it easier to balance yourself. It will also improve your overall handstand shape.

» If you are doing this exercise with your front facing the wall, it may be harder to come out of the handstand by turning to the side. Instead, try rolling forward out of the handstand.

Muscles Worked

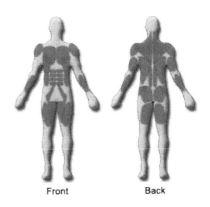

Front: Pectorals, Front Deltoids, Wrist Flexors, Abdominals, Obliques, Serratus, Hip Flexors, Hip Adductors, Quads

Back: Rear Deltoids, Rotator Cuff, Triceps, Wrist Extensors, Trapezius, Lats, Rhomboids, Lower Back, Gluteus Maximus, Hip Abductors, Hamstrings

Front   Back

Handstand: Arms Forward Lv1

Difficulty: ★★★☆☆

Directions

Stand with your back to a wall. Place your hands on the ground near your feet, then walk your feet up the wall into a handstand against the wall. Keeping your feet on the wall and your hands in place, let your shoulders move a few inches away from the wall so your arms are no longer perpendicular to the ground.

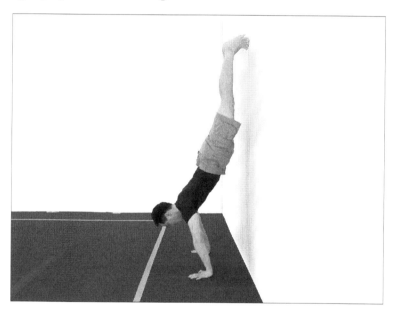

Comments

Leaning your shoulders away from the wall works your arms and shoulders in a different way than a regular handstand. Since your body will be at an angle, you will need to focus on your core muscles to keep it from arching.

Tips

» If you feel a lot of stress in your wrists from the forward lean, you can try turning your hands out to the sides.

Advanced
Progressions

Handstand: Arms Forward Lv1

Muscles Worked

Front: Pectorals, Front Deltoids, Biceps, Wrist Flexors, Abdominals, Obliques, Serratus, Hip Flexors, Hip Adductors, Quads

Back: Rear Deltoids, Rotator Cuff, Triceps, Wrist Extensors, Trapezius, Lats, Rhomboids, Lower Back, Gluteus Maximus, Hip Abductors, Hamstrings

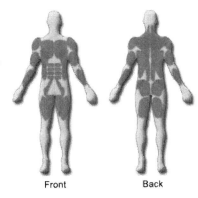

Front   Back

Handstand: Arms Forward Lv2

Difficulty: ★★★✬☆

Directions

Stand with your back to a wall. Place your hands on the ground about one-and-a-half to two feet in front of your feet, then walk your feet up the wall into a slanted handstand against the wall. Keeping your feet on the wall and hands in place, let your shoulders move ahead of your hands as far as they can. Your arms should no longer be perpendicular to the ground.

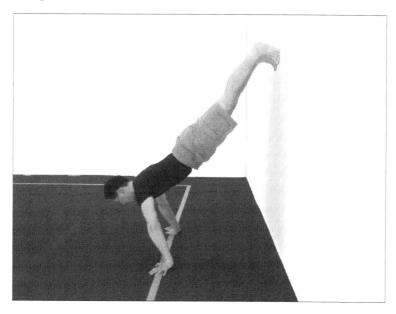

Comments

This exercise increases the forward lean of the shoulders more than the previous one. Again, your body will be at an angle, so you will need to focus on your core muscles to keep it from arching.

Tips

» If you feel a lot of stress in your wrists from the forward lean, you can try turning your hands out to the sides.

Advanced Progressions

Handstand: Arms Forward Lv2

Muscles Worked

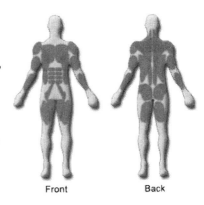

Front
Back

Front: Pectorals, Front Deltoids, Biceps, Wrist Flexors, Abdominals, Obliques, Serratus, Hip Flexors, Hip Adductors, Quads

Back: Rear Deltoids, Rotator Cuff, Triceps, Wrist Extensors, Trapezius, Lats, Rhomboids, Lower Back, Gluteus Maximus, Hip Abductors, Hamstrings

Handstand: Arms Forward Lv3

Difficulty: ★★★★☆

Directions

Stand with your back to a wall. Place your hands on the ground about three to four feet in front of your feet, then walk your feet up the wall into a slanted handstand against the wall. Keeping your feet on the wall and hands in place, let your shoulders move ahead of your hands as far as they can. Your arms should no longer be perpendicular to the ground.

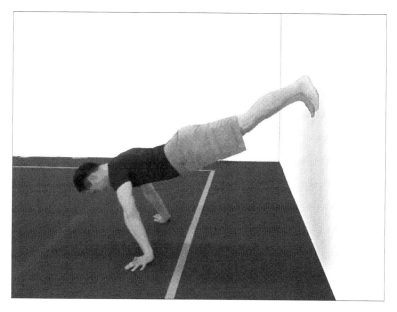

Comments

This exercise approaches the full planche position. However, since your body is not fully horizontal and your feet are on a wall, it is not nearly as difficult. That being said, this exercise will work intensely on the shoulders, arms, chest, and the core.

Tips

»   If you feel a lot of stress in your wrists from the forward lean, you can try turning your hands out to the sides.

Advanced Progressions

Handstand: Arms Forward Lv3

Muscles Worked

Front: Pectorals, Front Deltoids, Biceps, Wrist Flexors, Abdominals, Obliques, Serratus, Hip Flexors, Hip Adductors, Quads

Back: Rear Deltoids, Rotator Cuff, Triceps, Wrist Extensors, Trapezius, Lats, Rhomboids, Lower Back, Gluteus Maximus, Hip Abductors, Hamstrings

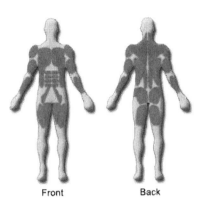

Front   Back

29

Front Levers

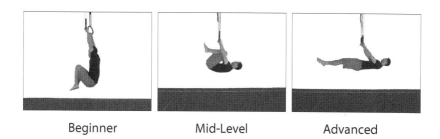

| Beginner | Mid-Level | Advanced |

The Front Lever Progression is a highly effective set of exercises that will work your entire body and build tremendous strength. That being said, this progression is more difficult than the basic ones. By the time you have mastered the advanced exercises in this progression, you will have an extremely strong core, which will be of great help in any activity that you do.

Since this progression involves pulling movements, your biceps, lats, and other pulling muscles will develop great strength. Your rotator cuff muscles will also be strengthened and your grip will improve. When performed correctly, these exercises strengthen the muscles that stabilize the shoulder joint, which can help improve weaknesses in your shoulder and reduce risk of injury in the future. In addition, you will learn how to properly hold your body during any activity that requires hanging from a support.

It is extremely important to focus on proper form in these exercises. It is relatively easy to perform the earlier exercises with poor form and think you have mastered them. However, when you move on to the advanced exercises, you will find yourself ill-prepared to perform them. Furthermore, poor form on these exercises means the muscles that stabilize the shoulder joint will not be strengthened as much as they could have been.

You can also do pull-ups in the Tuck Front Lever and more advanced exercises. Doing front lever pull-up variations will help increase your strength even faster. The key to doing pull-ups in any of the front lever positions is remembering to pull the bar or rings down toward your hips, not your chest. This will allow you to maintain your balance. If you pull the bar to your chest, your balance will be thrown off, and you will come down out of the front lever.

Equipment Needed

Pull-up bar or other suitably stable support to pull from with enough clearance from the wall for horizontal body work

Exercise Map

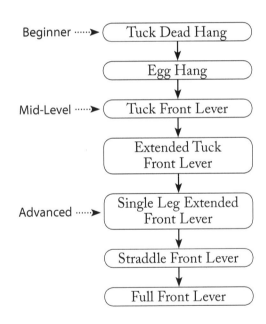

Beginner ·····▶ Tuck Dead Hang

Egg Hang

Mid-Level ·····▶ Tuck Front Lever

Extended Tuck Front Lever

Advanced ·····▶ Single Leg Extended Front Lever

Straddle Front Lever

Full Front Lever

Tuck Dead Hang

Difficulty: ★☆☆☆☆

Directions

Hang from the support with your knees tucked up toward your chest. Be sure to engage your shoulder girdle muscles so that you are pulling your shoulders tightly down into their sockets.

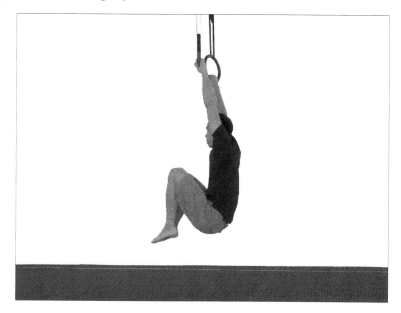

Comments

This exercise will prepare your grip and shoulder muscles, including the rotator cuff, for the later exercises. It will also work on your abs and hip flexors.

Tuck Dead Hang

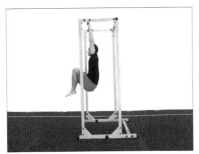

Pull-Up Bar Side View

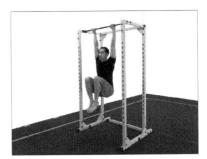

Pull-Up Bar Oblique View

Muscles Worked

Front: Front Deltoids, Biceps, Grip Muscles, Abdominals, Serratus, Hip Flexors

Back: Rear Deltoids, Rotator Cuff, Trapezius, Lats, Rhomboids, Lower Back

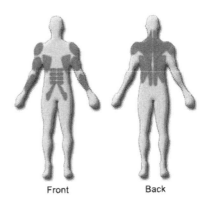

Front   Back

Egg Hang

Difficulty: ★☆☆☆☆

Directions

Hang from the support with your knees tucked up toward your chest. At the shoulders, pull your body forward and up so that your chest forms a 45-degree angle with the floor. Make sure your arms are straight and you are engaging your shoulder girdle muscles so that your shoulders are pulled tightly down into their sockets.

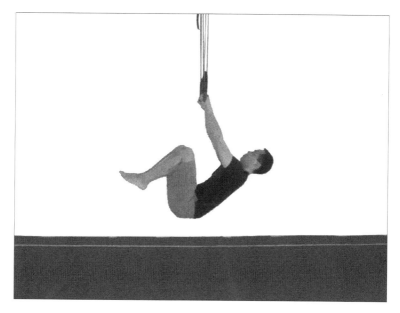

Comments

This is the first exercise to work on front lever movement. You will be working on all of the major muscles in your upper body, including the pectorals, trapezius, lats, rhomboids, rotator cuff, and arm muscles. Tucking the legs makes the lever movement easier by reducing the amount of reverse leverage.

Tips

» It is very important to keep your elbows straight, or you will not work the target muscles as effectively. While easier, bending your elbows will slow your progress to the more advanced exercises.

Advanced Progressions

Egg Hang

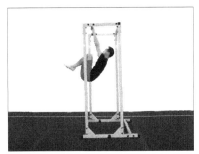

Pull-Up Bar Side View

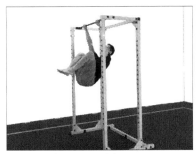

Pull-Up Bar Oblique View

Muscles Worked

Front: Pectorals, Biceps, Grip Muscles, Wrist Flexors, Abdominals, Serratus, Hip Flexors

Back: Rear Deltoids, Rotator Cuff, Triceps, Trapezius, Lats, Rhomboids, Lower Back

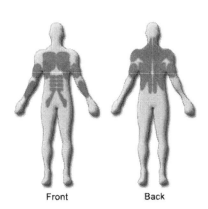

Front   Back

Tuck Front Lever

Difficulty: ★★☆☆☆

Directions

Hang from the support with your knees tucked up to your chest and your back rounded. At the shoulders, pull your body forward and up so that your upper body is horizontal. Be sure to engage your shoulder girdle muscles so that your shoulders are pulled tightly down into their sockets. Remember to keep your arms straight.

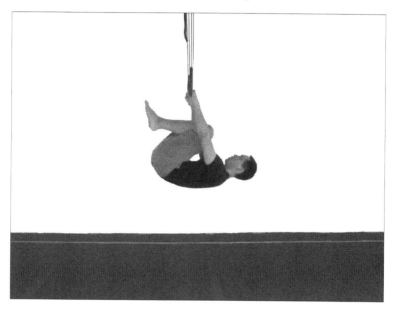

Comments

This exercise puts your upper body in the fully horizontal position of a front lever. You will need to contract your lats and engage your chest muscles to maintain stability.

Tips

» Focus on pushing the bar (or whatever support you are hanging from) down toward your feet. This will assist in keeping your torso horizontal.

» Even though your legs are tucked, you will need to contract your core in order to maintain the horizontal position.

» Don't forget to breathe! If you find yourself holding your breath, try taking shallow breaths.

» It is very important to keep your elbows straight, or you will not work the target muscles as effectively. While easier, bending your elbows will slow your progress to the more advanced exercises.

» As you get tired, you may be tempted to relax your shoulder muscles, letting your shoulders move forward in their sockets. Avoid doing this, as it can be dangerous for your shoulder joints. Focus on contracting your shoulder blades together to prevent this from happening.

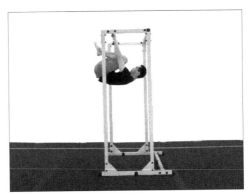

Pull-Up Bar Side View

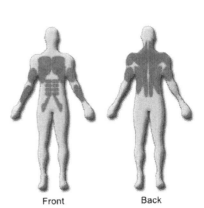

Muscles Worked

Front: Pectorals, Biceps, Grip Muscles, Wrist Flexors, Abdominals, Serratus, Hip Flexors

Back: Rear Deltoids, Rotator Cuff, Triceps, Trapezius, Lats, Rhomboids, Lower Back

Front   Back

Extended Tuck Front Lever

Difficulty: ★★☆☆☆

Directions

Hang from the support with your knees tucked up, but with your back straight and extended. At the shoulders, pull your body forward and up so that your upper body is horizontal. Be sure to engage your shoulder girdle muscles so that your shoulders are pulled tightly down into their sockets. Remember to keep your arms straight.

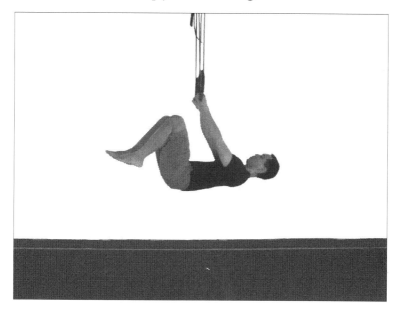

Comments

This exercise is similar to the previous one, but instead of rounding your back, keep it straight. While this may seem like a small difference, it makes the exercise significantly harder by increasing the amount of reverse leverage. You will need to contract your lats even more and engage your chest muscles to maintain stability.

Tips

» Focus on pushing the bar (or whatever support you are hanging from) down toward your feet. This will assist in keeping your torso horizontal.

» Even though your legs are tucked, you will need to contract your core in order to maintain the horizontal position.

» Don't forget to breathe! If you find yourself holding your breath, try taking shallow breaths.

» It is very important to keep your elbows straight, or you will not work the target muscles as effectively. While easier, bending your elbows will slow your progress to the more advanced exercises.

» As you get tired, you may be tempted to relax your shoulder muscles, letting your shoulders move forward in their sockets. Avoid doing this, as it can be dangerous for your shoulder joints. Focus on contracting your shoulder blades together to prevent this from happening.

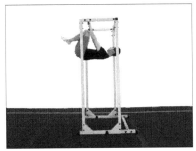

Pull-Up Bar Side View

Muscles Worked

Front: Pectorals, Biceps, Grip Muscles, Wrist Flexors, Abdominals, Obliques, Serratus, Hip Flexors, Hip Adductors

Back: Rear Deltoids, Rotator Cuff, Triceps, Trapezius, Lats, Rhomboids, Lower Back, Gluteus Maximus, Hip Abductors

Front   Back

Advanced
Progressions

Single Leg Extended Front Lever

Difficulty: ★★★☆☆

Directions

Enter the Extended Tuck Front Lever position, then extend one leg so that it is parallel to the ground. Keep the other leg in a tucked position.

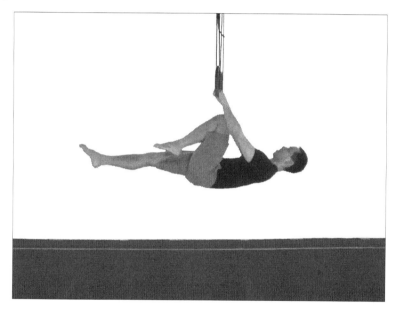

Comments

Extending just one leg makes this exercise much harder than the previous one. You will need to contract your core intensely in order to keep the body straight.

Tips

» If it is too difficult at first, you can try tucking the bent leg even tighter to the chest. This will help reduce the load on the target muscles. Alternatively, you can bend the extended leg slightly to decrease the reverse leverage a bit. However, be sure to keep your body as horizontal as you can.

» Don't forget to breathe! If you find yourself holding your breath, try taking shallow breaths.

» It is very important to keep your elbows straight, or you will not work the target muscles as effectively. While easier, bending your elbows will slow your progress to the more advanced exercises.

» As you get tired, you may be tempted to relax your shoulder muscles, letting your shoulders move forward in their sockets. Avoid doing this, as it can be dangerous for your shoulder joints. Focus on contracting your shoulder blades together to prevent this from happening.

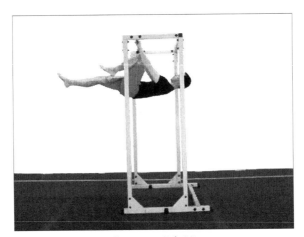

Pull-Up Bar Side View

Muscles Worked

Front: Pectorals, Biceps, Grip Muscles, Wrist Flexors, Abdominals, Obliques, Serratus, Hip Flexors, Hip Adductors, Quads

Back: Rear Deltoids, Rotator Cuff, Triceps, Trapezius, Lats, Rhomboids, Lower Back, Gluteus Maximus, Hip Abductors, Hamstrings

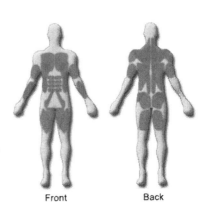

Front   Back

Straddle Front Lever

Difficulty: ★★★★☆

Directions

Enter the Extended Tuck Front Lever position, then extend both legs into a horizontal straddle position.

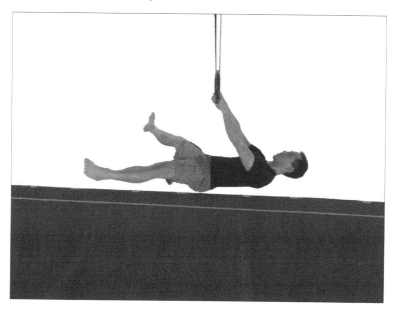

Comments

This exercise utilizes a straddle position, which may be difficult if your hip flexors are not used to it. It will require a lot of core strength to maintain this position. Be sure to keep your legs in line with your upper body, which should be parallel to the ground.

Tips

» You'll have to push the support even harder toward your feet while intensely contracting your core at the same time.

» Don't forget to breathe! If you find yourself holding your breath, try taking shallow breaths.

» It is very important to keep your elbows straight, or you will not work the target muscles as effectively. While easier, bending your elbows will slow your progress to the more advanced exercises.

» As you get tired, you may be tempted to relax your shoulder muscles, letting your shoulders move forward in their sockets. Avoid doing this, as it can be dangerous for your shoulder joints. Focus on contracting your shoulder blades together to prevent this from happening.

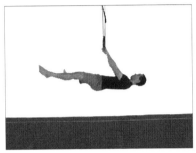

Alternate Rings Side View

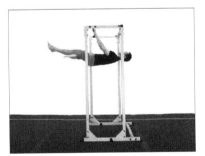

Pull-Up Bar Side View

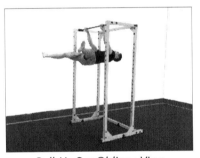

Pull-Up Bar Oblique View

Muscles Worked

Front: Pectorals, Biceps, Grip Muscles, Wrist Flexors, Abdominals, Obliques, Serratus, Hip Flexors, Hip Adductors, Quads

Back: Rear Deltoids, Rotator Cuff, Triceps, Trapezius, Lats, Rhomboids, Lower Back, Gluteus Maximus, Hip Abductors, Hamstrings

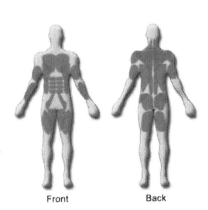

Front   Back

Full Front Lever

Difficulty: ★★★★★

Directions

Enter the Extended Tuck Front Lever position, then extend both legs so that they are horizontal and together.

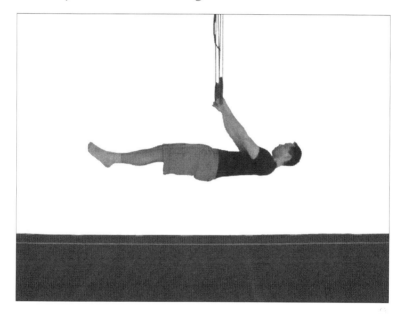

Comments

This is an extremely difficult exercise to do well. Contract your entire body intensely so that each muscle group can use its antagonist to help maintain your body position.

Tips

» Like the previous exercises, remember to breathe and keep your elbows straight. Remember to contract your shoulder blades together, and don't let your shoulder muscles relax at any time.

Advanced
Progressions

Full Front Lever

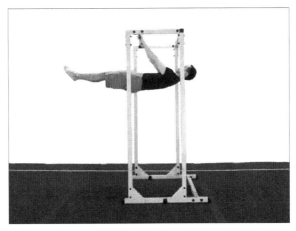

Pull-Up Bar Side View

Muscles Worked

Front: Pectorals, Biceps, Grip Muscles, Wrist Flexors, Abdominals, Obliques, Serratus, Hip Flexors, Hip Adductors, Quads

Back: Rear Deltoids, Rotator Cuff, Triceps, Trapezius, Lats, Rhomboids, Lower Back, Gluteus Maximus, Hip Abductors, Hamstrings

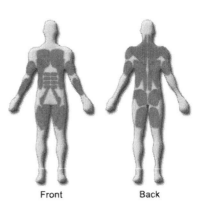

Front   Back

30

Back Levers

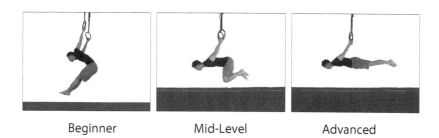

| Beginner | Mid-Level | Advanced |

The Back Lever Progression provides an excellent full-body workout and develops an extraordinarily strong core. A back lever does not require as much strength as a front lever, but the position will take some time to get used to. There is a component of shoulder flexibility involved in these exercises as well, but the role it plays gets smaller as you advance through the progression.

Since this progression involves pulling movements, your biceps, lats, and rotator cuff muscles will be targeted. Also, since your arms are behind you, your chest muscles will be worked in a pulling motion as well. When performed correctly, these exercises strengthen the muscles that stabilize the shoulder joint, which can help improve weaknesses in your shoulder and reduce the risk of injury in the future. In addition, you will learn how to properly hold your body during any activity that requires hanging from a support.

It is extremely important to focus on proper form in these exercises. It is relatively easy to perform the earlier exercises with poor form and think you have mastered them. However, when you move on to the advanced exercises, you will find yourself ill-prepared to perform them. Furthermore, poor form on these exercises means the muscles that stabilize the shoulder joint will not be strengthened as much as they could have been.

Equipment Needed

Pull-up bar or other suitably stable support to pull from, and enough clearance from the wall for horizontal body work

Exercise Map

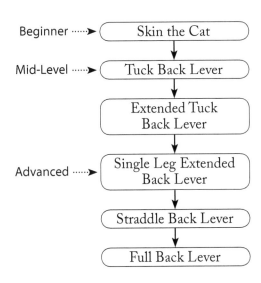

Skin the Cat

Difficulty: ★☆☆☆☆

Directions

Hang from the support with your knees tucked up to your chest. Rotate your body up, putting your feet between your arms (and under the support if using a bar). Keep going until your feel a stretch in your shoulders, then let your legs hang down. Be sure to keep your shoulder muscles engaged the entire time, even when you are just hanging in the final position.

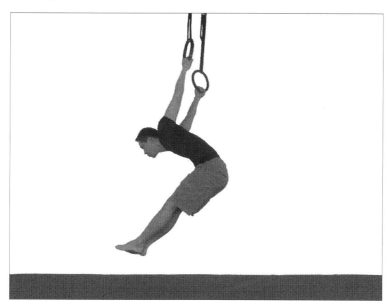

Comments

While this exercise is not a back lever, it will prepare you for later exercises. It is similar to a move you may have done on the monkey bars when you were a kid. How far you can hang down depends on your shoulder flexibility. Go as far as is comfortable and then engage your muscles to maintain the position. You should feel a good stretch in the shoulders. If you start feeling pain, then you have gone too far and should come out of the position. If you have very flexible shoulders, you will probably be hanging almost vertically. On the other hand, if you have tight shoulders, your upper body will probably be just below horizontal.

Tips

» Contract the muscles in your chest, shoulders, upper back, and lats to stabilize your position. Your chest muscles will help counteract gravity, which is trying to pull you down and rotate your shoulders further. Your upper back will help maintain your upper body in a rigid position so that your chest muscles have something to work off of.

» You can come out of the position by either going back the way you came, or carefully letting go of the support and landing on your feet.

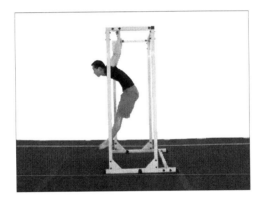

Pull-Up Bar Side View

Muscles Worked

Front: Pectorals, Front Deltoids, Biceps, Grip Muscles, Serratus

Back: Rotator Cuff, Trapezius, Lats, Rhomboids

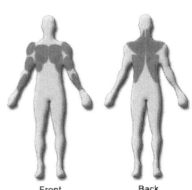

Front   Back

Tuck Back Lever

Difficulty: ★☆☆☆☆

Directions

Hang from the bar with your knees tucked up to your chest. Rotate your body up, putting your feet between your arms (and under the support if you are using a bar). Keep going until your chest is horizontal. Keep your back rounded and your knees tucked up under your torso. Be sure to keep your shoulder muscles engaged.

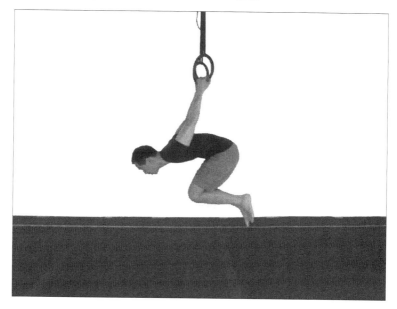

Comments

This is the first exercise in the actual back lever position. It may take a while to get used to it.

Tips

» When going into the position, you may not immediately know just how far to rotate before reaching the horizontal position. It may help to have a mirror around, or have a friend tell you if your upper body is horizontal.

» Think about pressing the support down toward your feet to help maintain the position. Even though your legs are tucked, you will need to contract your core to maintain the horizontal position.

» Don't forget to breathe! If you find yourself holding your breath, try taking shallow breaths.

» As you get tired, you may be tempted to relax your shoulder muscles and let your shoulders move backward in their sockets. Avoid doing this, as it can be dangerous for your shoulder joints. Prevent this by focusing on squeezing your shoulders together toward the front.

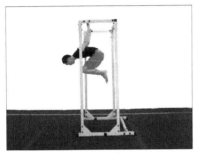
Pull-Up Bar Side View

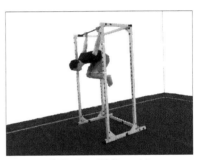
Pull-Up Bar Oblique View

Muscles Worked

Front: Pectorals, Front Deltoids, Biceps, Grip Muscles, Wrist Flexors, Abdominals, Obliques, Serratus

Back: Rear Deltoids, Rotator Cuff, Triceps, Trapezius, Lats, Rhomboids, Hamstrings

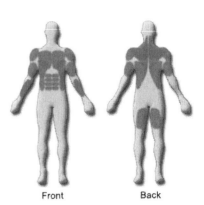

Front   Back

Advanced Progressions

Extended Tuck Back Lever

Difficulty: ★★☆☆☆

Directions

Hang from the support with your knees tucked up to your chest. Rotate your body up, putting your feet between your arms (and under the support if you are using a bar). Keep going until your chest is horizontal. Keep your knees in a tucked position, but extend your lower back so that it is straight instead of rounded. Be sure to keep your shoulder muscles engaged.

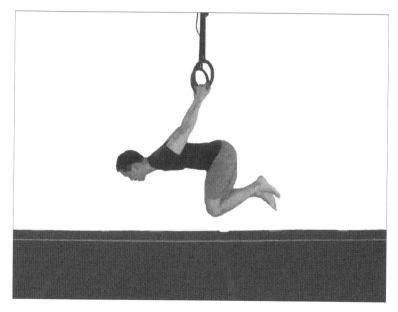

Comments

This exercise is similar to the previous one, but instead of rounding the lower back, it is kept straight. While this may seem like a small difference, it makes the exercise significantly harder by increasing reverse leverage. You will need to contract your chest to counteract this leverage, while engaging your lats and upper back muscles to maintain stability.

Tips

» Focus on pushing the bar (or the support you are hanging from) down toward your feet. Even though your legs are tucked, you will need to contract your core intensely to maintain the horizontal position.

» Don't forget to breathe! If you find yourself holding your breath, try taking shallow breaths.

» As you get tired, you may be tempted to relax your shoulder muscles and let your shoulders move backward in their sockets. Avoid doing this, as it can be dangerous for your shoulder joints. Prevent this by focusing on squeezing your shoulders together toward the front.

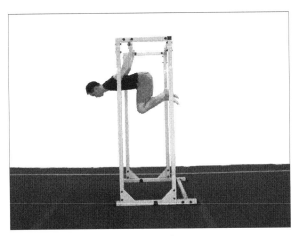

Pull-Up Bar Side View

Muscles Worked

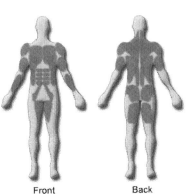

Front: Pectorals, Front Deltoids, Biceps, Grip Muscles, Wrist Flexors, Abdominals, Obliques, Serratus, Hip Flexors, Hip Adductors

Back: Rear Deltoids, Rotator Cuff, Triceps, Trapezius, Lats, Rhomboids, Lower Back, Gluteus Maximus, Hip Abductors, Hamstrings

Front   Back

Advanced Progressions

Single Leg Extended Back Lever

Difficulty: ★★★☆☆

Directions

Hang from the support with your knees tucked up to your chest. Rotate your body up, putting your feet between your arms (and under the support if using a bar). Keep going until your chest is horizontal. Keep one knee in a tucked position and extend the other leg out so that it is horizontal and in line with your upper body. Be sure to keep your shoulder muscles engaged.

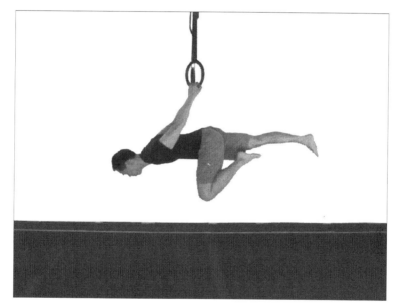

Comments

Extending just one leg makes this exercise much harder than the previous one due to increased reverse leverage.

Tips

» If it is too difficult at first, you can try tucking the bent leg even tighter toward the chest. This will help reduce the load on the target muscles. You will need to contract your core intensely, but try not to arch your back.

» Alternatively, you can bend your extended leg at the knee a little bit. However, keep the thigh horizontal and in line with your upper body. This way, you can reduce the load on the target muscles without losing the extended position in the hips.

» Don't forget to breathe! If you find yourself holding your breath, try taking shallow breaths.

» As you get tired, you may be tempted to relax your shoulder muscles and let your shoulders move backward in their sockets. Avoid doing this, as it can be dangerous for your shoulder joints. Prevent this by focusing on squeezing your shoulders together toward the front.

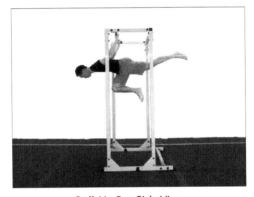

Pull-Up Bar Side View

Muscles Worked

Front: Pectorals, Front Deltoids, Biceps, Grip Muscles, Wrist Flexors, Abdominals, Obliques, Serratus, Hip Flexors, Hip Adductors, Quads

Back: Rear Deltoids, Rotator Cuff, Triceps, Trapezius, Lats, Rhomboids, Lower Back, Gluteus Maximus, Hip Abductors, Hamstrings

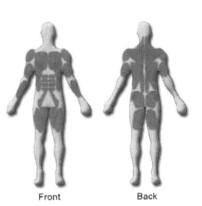

Front   Back

Straddle Back Lever

Difficulty: ★★★✬☆

Directions

Hang from the support with your knees tucked up to your chest. Rotate your body up, putting your feet between your arms (and under the support if using a bar). Keep going until your chest is horizontal. Extend both legs out in a straddle position so that they are parallel to the ground. Be sure to keep your shoulder muscles engaged.

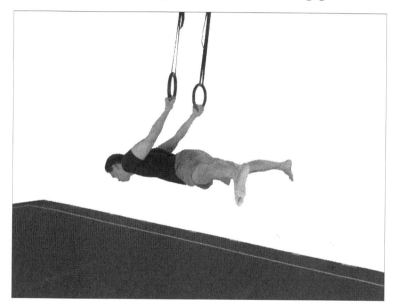

Comments

This exercise utilizes a straddle position, which may be difficult if your hip abductors are not used to it. It will require a lot of core strength to maintain this position. Try not to arch the back or bend the legs, even though that makes it feel easier. In the long run, doing so will slow your progress to the next exercise. Be sure to keep your legs in line with your upper body, which should be parallel to the ground.

Tips

» You will have to push the support even harder toward your feet.

Advanced Progressions

» Don't forget to breathe! If you find yourself holding your breath, try taking shallow breaths.

» As you get tired, you may be tempted to relax your shoulder muscles and let your shoulders move backward in their sockets. Avoid doing this, as it can be dangerous for your shoulder joints. Prevent this by focusing on squeezing your shoulders together toward the front.

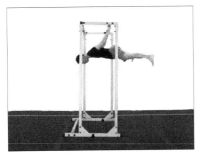

Pull-Up Bar Side View

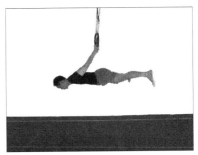

Alternate Rings Side View

Muscles Worked

Front: Pectorals, Front Deltoids, Biceps, Grip Muscles, Wrist Flexors, Abdominals, Obliques, Serratus, Hip Flexors, Hip Adductors, Quads

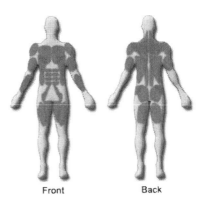

Front   Back

Back: Rear Deltoids, Rotator Cuff, Triceps, Trapezius, Lats, Rhomboids, Lower Back, Gluteus Maximus, Hip Abductors, Hamstrings

Advanced
Progressions

Full Back Lever

Difficulty: ★★★★☆

Directions

Hang from the support with your knees tucked up to your chest. Rotate your body up, putting your feet between your arms (and under the support if using a bar). Keep going until your chest is horizontal. Extend both legs out so that they are together and horizontal. Be sure to keep your shoulder muscles engaged.

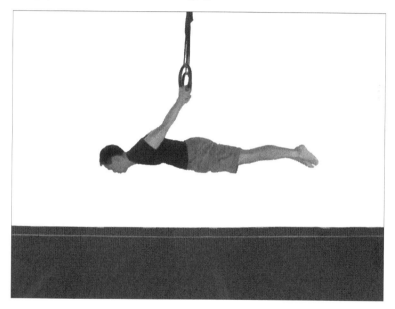

Comments

This is an extremely difficult exercise to do well. Contract your entire body intensely so that each muscle group can use its antagonist to help maintain your body position.

Tips

» As in the previous exercises, remember to breathe and try not to arch your back.

» Do not let your shoulder muscles relax! Remember to squeeze your shoulders together in the front.

Advanced Progressions

Full Back Lever

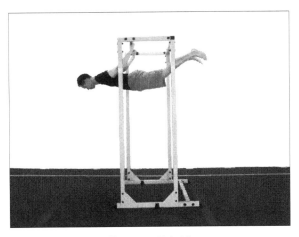

Pull-Up Bar Side View
Try to keep the legs horizontal, instead
of arched as shown in this picture.

Muscles Worked

Front: Pectorals, Front Deltoids, Biceps, Grip Muscles, Wrist Flexors, Abdominals, Obliques, Serratus, Hip Flexors, Hip Adductors, Quads

Back: Rear Deltoids, Rotator Cuff, Triceps, Trapezius, Lats, Rhomboids, Lower Back, Gluteus Maximus, Hip Abductors, Hamstrings

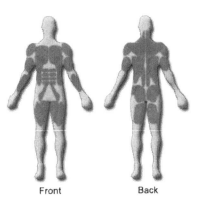

Front   Back

31

Pull-Ups

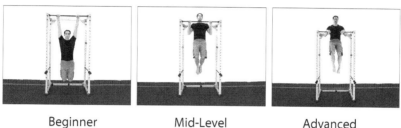

| Beginner | Mid-Level | Advanced |

Pull-Ups and Chin-Ups are great upper body exercises that work many muscle groups. If you have never been able to do one, this progression will help you get there. If you are already able to do a few, you will be able to do many more in a row by the time you are done with this progression. If pull-ups are too easy for you, this progression will help you move on to the slow muscle-up, which requires both great pulling and pushing strength.

There are two common grips used for these exercises. Overhand grips are used for pull-ups and underhand grips are used for chin-ups. In the overhand grip, you grip the bar with your palms facing away from you. In the underhand grip, your palms face you. They work on your muscles in slightly different ways, and most people will find one easier than the other. Which one is easier depends on what you feel is more natural. For the beginning exercises, it is a good idea to work on both types of grips. However, for the later ones, the overhand grip is recommended, as it will be more difficult to push at the top of a pull-up using an underhand grip. While it is possible to use an underhand grip for dynamic exercises, maintaining a static position with that grip will not give you much functional benefit.

Equipment Needed

Pull-up bar or other suitably stable support to pull from

Exercise Map

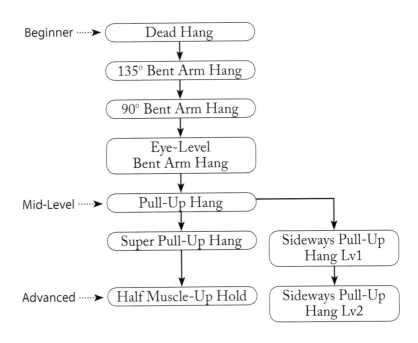

Dead Hang

Difficulty: ★☆☆☆☆

Directions

Place your hands on the bar and hang with your body straight down and your feet off the ground. Be sure to keep your shoulders engaged (pulled down away from your ears), especially when you get tired.

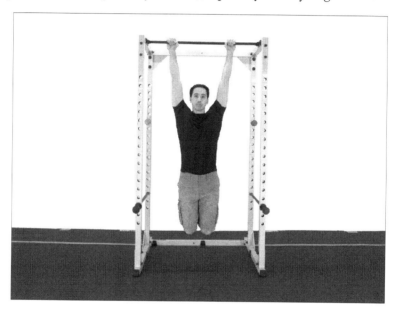

Comments

This exercise will build your grip strength as well as necessary shoulder strength to hang safely. It is extremely important to keep your shoulders engaged, or your entire body weight will be placed on your shoulder ligaments. By engaging your shoulders, you will strengthen the muscles that help stabilize the shoulder joint, including the rotator cuff.

Dead Hang

Muscles Worked

Front: Front Deltoids, Biceps, Grip Muscles

Back: Rear Deltoids, Rotator Cuff, Trapezius, Lats, Rhomboids

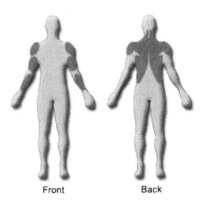

Front   Back

135° Bent Arm Hang

Difficulty: ★☆☆☆☆

Directions

From a dead hang on the bar, pull your body up and hold your position when your elbows reach a 135-degree angle.

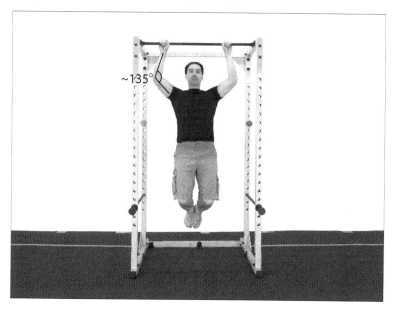

Comments

This exercise will start building your upper body pulling strength. Focus on pulling with your biceps as well as your lats and upper back muscles.

Tips

» Squeezing your shoulder blades down and together can help you better engage your upper back muscles.

135° Bent Arm Hang

Muscles Worked

Front: Pectorals, Front Deltoids, Biceps, Grip Muscles, Abdominals, Obliques, Serratus

Back: Rear Deltoids, Rotator Cuff, Trapezius, Lats, Rhomboids

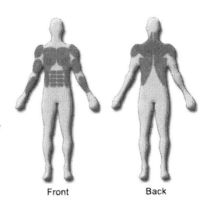

Front   Back

90° Bent Arm Hang

Difficulty: ★⯪☆☆☆

Directions

From a dead hang on the bar, pull your body up and hold your position when your elbows reach a 90-degree angle. The bar will be near the top of your head.

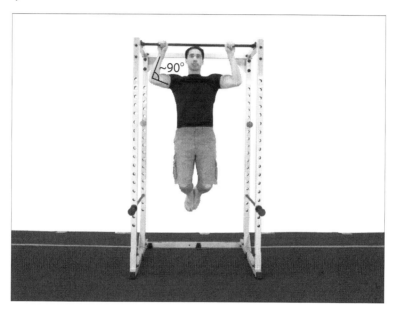

Comments

Remember to focus on pulling with your biceps as well as your lats and upper back muscles. As your body gets closer to the bar, the effort will shift from the biceps to the lats.

Tips

» Squeezing your shoulder blades down and together can help you better engage your upper back muscles.

90° Bent Arm Hang

Muscles Worked

Front: Pectorals, Front Deltoids, Biceps, Grip Muscles, Abdominals, Obliques, Serratus

Back: Rear Deltoids, Rotator Cuff, Trapezius, Lats, Rhomboids

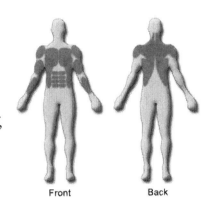

Front   Back

Eye-Level Bent Arm Hang

Difficulty: ★★☆☆☆

Directions

From a dead hang on the bar, pull your body up and hold your position when the bar reaches eye level. Your elbows will be at about a 45-degree angle.

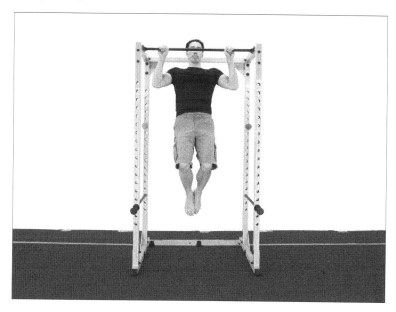

Comments

Remember to focus on pulling with your biceps as well as your lats and upper back muscles. As your body gets closer to the bar, the effort will shift from the biceps to the lats.

Tips

» Squeezing your shoulder blades down and together can help you better engage your upper back muscles.

Eye-Level Bent Arm Hang

Muscles Worked

Front: Pectorals, Front Deltoids, Biceps, Grip Muscles, Abdominals, Obliques, Serratus

Back: Rear Deltoids, Rotator Cuff, Trapezius, Lats, Rhomboids

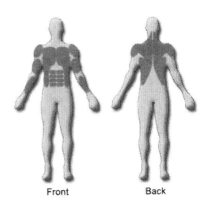

Front   Back

Pull-Up Hang

Difficulty: ★★✬☆☆

Directions

From a dead hang on the bar, pull your body up and hold with the bar just below your chin.

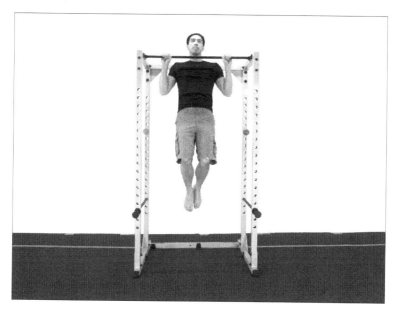

Comments

You should be engaging your lats and upper back muscles intensely.

Tips

» Squeezing your shoulder blades down and together can help you better engage your upper back muscles more strongly.

Pull-Up Hang

Muscles Worked

Front: Pectorals, Front Deltoids, Biceps, Grip Muscles, Abdominals, Obliques, Serratus

Back: Rear Deltoids, Rotator Cuff, Trapezius, Lats, Rhomboids

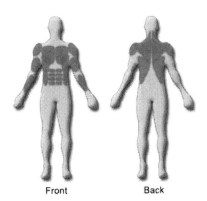

Front   Back

Super Pull-Up Hang

Difficulty: ★★★☆☆

Directions

From a dead hang on the bar, pull your body up and hold with the bar at the level of your chest.

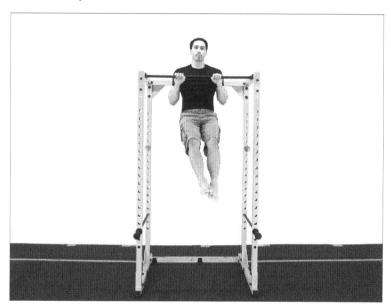

Comments

This exercise starts introducing a pushing component, which can be quite difficult at first. It is critical to engage your upper back, lats, and chest muscles so that your arms have a rigid body to push up. This exercise will help with the transition portion of the muscle-up.

Tips

» An overhand grip is recommended for this exercise due to the pushing component. You can use a normal grip or you can try using a false grip on the bar. The false grip will make the pushing component easier, since it essentially shortens your arm and lets you push from the wrist. A normal grip is more difficult, because you will be pushing from the hands, which are farther from the body than the wrists. You will also need to keep the wrists as rigid as possible to transfer the pushing power to the bar effectively. Finally, you'll need good grip strength to prevent your hands from rotating down as you push.

» To use a false grip on the bar, place your wrists on top of the bar with the base of the hand touching the bar. Next, rotate your hands inward a bit so that you can grip the bar with the rest of your hand and fingers. It will feel awkward at first, but eventually you'll get used to it.

Muscles Worked

Front: Pectorals, Biceps, Grip Muscles, Abdominals, Obliques, Serratus

Back: Rear Deltoids, Rotator Cuff, Triceps, Trapezius, Lats, Rhomboids

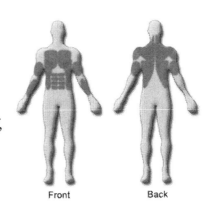

Front   Back

Half Muscle-Up Hold

Difficulty: ★★★★☆

Directions

From a dead hang on the bar, pull your body up to your chest, then start pushing down so that your body continues moving up. Hold your position when the bar is right below your rib cage. Your elbows should be bent to near 90 degrees.

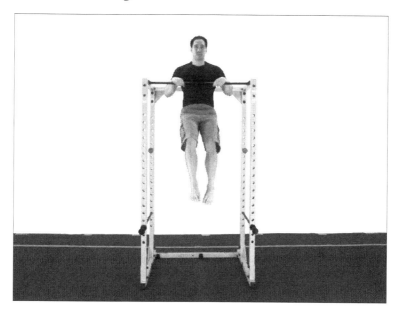

Comments

This exercise is similar to the end of the transition portion of a muscle-up. It works mostly on your pushing strength.

Tips

» A false grip is recommended for this exercise, since you'll be pushing from a very difficult position. If you choose to use a normal overhand grip, you'll need to have exceptional grip strength. It will also help to grip the bar so that your wrists are near-horizontal, rather than hanging down as they would be for a traditional pull-up.

Half Muscle-Up Hold

Muscles Worked

Front: Pectorals, Front Deltoids, Abdominals, Obliques, Serratus

Back: Rear Deltoids, Rotator Cuff, Triceps, Trapezius, Lats, Rhomboids

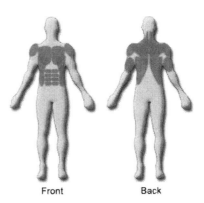

Front   Back

Sideways Pull-Up Hang Lv1

Difficulty: ★★★☆☆

Directions

From a dead hang on the bar, pull your body up so the bar is just below your chin. Next, move your body sideways, so the center of your body lines up with one of your hands.

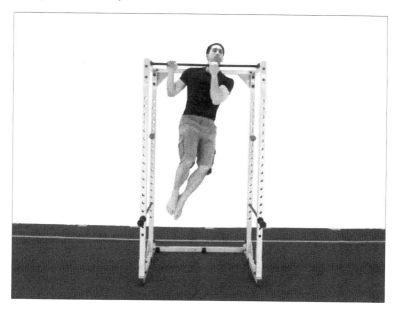

Comments

This exercise introduces asymmetry and will work one side of your body more intensely. Working the target muscles from different angles will improve your functional strength. You will need to use your upper back and chest muscles to help move your body to one side. This exercise will start giving you a sense of what an assisted one-arm pull-up feels like.

Advanced
Progressions

Sideways Pull-Up Hang Lv1

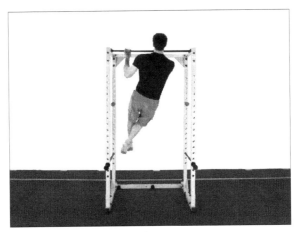

Back View

Muscles Worked

Front: Pectorals, Front Deltoids, Biceps, Grip Muscles, Abdominals, Obliques, Serratus

Back: Rear Deltoids, Rotator Cuff, Trapezius, Lats, Rhomboids

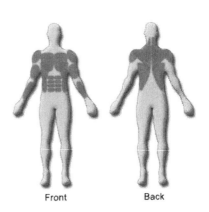

Front   Back

Sideways Pull-Up Hang Lv2

Difficulty: ★★★★☆

Directions

From a dead hang on the bar, pull your body up so the bar is just below your chin. Next, move your body sideways so that your shoulder is as close as possible to being in line with the opposite hand.

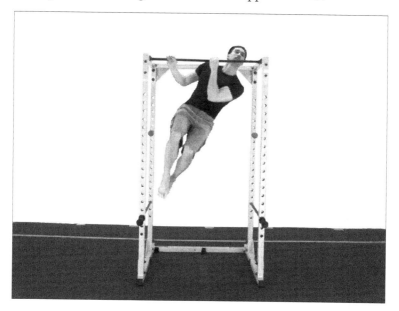

Comments

This exercise introduces even more asymmetry and will work one side of your body even more intensely. It will work the target muscles from different angles, which will further improve your functional strength. The balance of this exercise may be difficult at first, but it will get easier with time and increased strength.

Sideways Pull-Up Hang Lv2

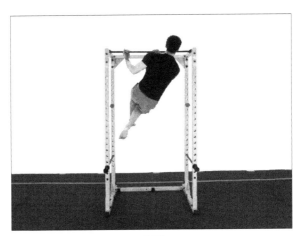

Back View

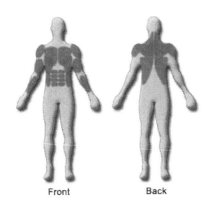

Front   Back

Muscles Worked

Front: Pectorals, Front Deltoids, Biceps, Grip Muscles, Abdominals, Obliques, Serratus

Back: Rear Deltoids, Rotator Cuff, Trapezius, Lats, Rhomboids

32

One-Arm Pull-Ups

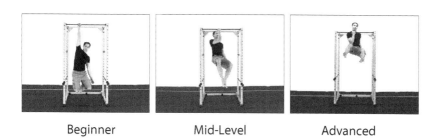

Beginner   Mid-Level   Advanced

One-Arm Pull-Ups and One-Arm Chin-Ups are no easy feat. Aside from obvious strength requirements, balancing your body while performing these one-sided movements is tricky. These exercises are very advanced and are for people looking to develop extreme strength. The ability to do regular two-armed pull-ups easily is a prerequisite, and the ability to do many of them in a row will be quite helpful. Satisfying this prerequisite means that you have developed adequate strength to hang and pull properly from a support with your hands.

As with a two-armed pull-up, you can split the movement into two different phases. The first phase utilizes both your biceps and lats with emphasis on your biceps. The second phase begins when your biceps have nearly reached full contraction so the rest of the movement is completed by your lats and upper back muscles.

Due to the one-sided nature of this movement, you will need to balance your body as you go through the pulling movement. This balance will change slightly depending on whether you use an overhand or underhand grip. Either way, you will find yourself trying to align your pulling hand with the center of your body. This generally means using your chest muscles to help turn your body toward the pulling arm. If you are not used to doing one-sided exercises, you might find yourself contracting the muscles of the other side as well. This does not help with the movement itself and should be avoided.

Since your entire body weight is being placed on a single arm, your muscles and joints will be under a lot of stress. Do not push yourself too hard or try to progress too quickly through these exercises. Give your body adequate time to adapt to these high levels of stress. Otherwise, you risk developing injuries like elbow tendonitis. In the event that you start developing pain when performing these exercises, stop doing them immediately. Let your body heal completely before resuming this progression. Depending on the nature and severity of the injury, it can take several weeks to months to fully recover. If the pain does not improve after stopping these exercises, consult your physician.

Equipment Needed

Pull-up bar or other suitably stable support to pull from

Exercise Map

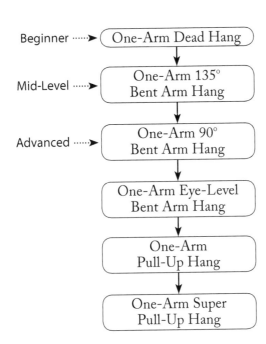

One-Arm Dead Hang

Difficulty: ★✫☆☆☆

Directions

Place one hand on the bar and hang with your body straight down and your feet off the ground. Be sure to keep your shoulder engaged (pulled down away from your ear), especially when you get tired.

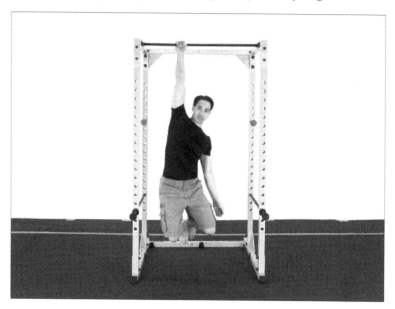

Comments

This exercise will work on your shoulder muscles so that you can safely hold your entire body weight on one arm. It will also develop your grip strength so that it does not become a limiting factor in these exercises.

Tips

» For overall strength development, it is a good idea to work on both overhand and underhand grips.

Advanced Progressions

One-Arm Dead Hang

Muscles Worked

Front: Front Deltoids, Biceps, Grip Muscles

Back: Rear Deltoids, Rotator Cuff, Trapezius, Lats, Rhomboids

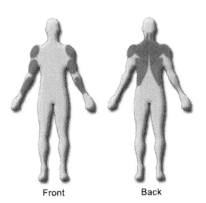

Front   Back

One-Arm 135° Bent Arm Hang

Difficulty: ★★✬☆☆

Directions

From a one-arm dead hang on the bar, pull your body up and hold your position when your elbow reaches a 135-degree angle.

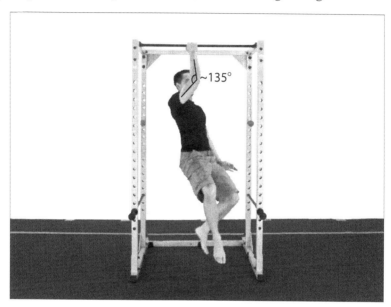

Comments

This exercise starts working on your one-arm pulling strength. You will need to engage the lats, upper back, and chest muscles to assist in the pull, as well as to help balance your body.

Tips

» For overall strength development, it is a good idea to work on both overhand and underhand grips. The overhand grip will place more stress on the elbow joint. If this grip is uncomfortable, stop using it and just use the underhand grip.

One-Arm 135° Bent Arm Hang

Muscles Worked

Front: Pectorals, Front Deltoids, Biceps, Grip Muscles, Abdominals, Obliques, Serratus

Back: Rear Deltoids, Rotator Cuff, Trapezius, Lats, Rhomboids

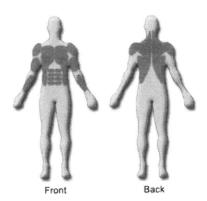

Front   Back

One-Arm 90° Bent Arm Hang

Difficulty: ★★★⯪☆

Directions

From a one-arm dead hang on the pull-up bar, pull your body up and hold your position when your elbow reaches a 90-degree angle. The bar will be around the top of your head.

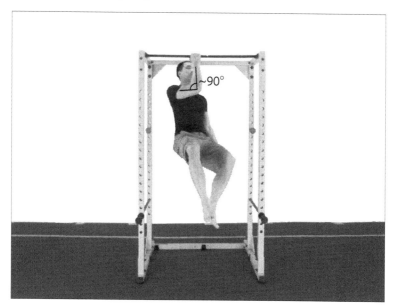

Comments

Remember to focus on pulling with your biceps as well as your lats and upper back muscles. The closer your body gets to the bar, the more the intensity will shift from the biceps to the lats.

Tips

» For overall strength development, it is a good idea to work on both overhand and underhand grips. The overhand grip will place more stress on the elbow joint. If this grip is uncomfortable, stop using it and just use the underhand grip.

One-Arm 90° Bent Arm Hang

Muscles Worked

Front: Pectorals, Front Deltoids, Biceps, Grip Muscles, Abdominals, Obliques, Serratus

Back: Rear Deltoids, Rotator Cuff, Trapezius, Lats, Rhomboids

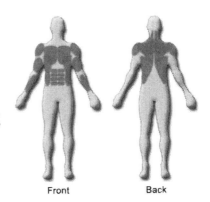

Front   Back

One-Arm Eye-Level Bent Arm Hang

Difficulty: ★★★★☆

Directions

From a one-arm dead hang on the bar, pull your body up and hold your position when the bar is at eye level. Your elbow will be between 90 degrees and 45 degrees.

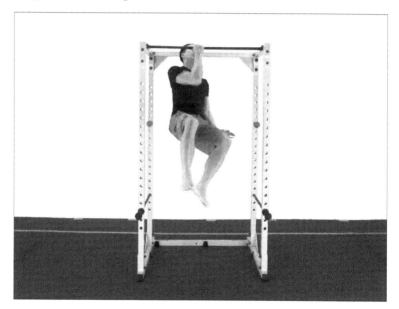

Comments

Remember to focus on pulling with your biceps as well as your lats and upper back muscles. The closer your body gets to the bar, the more the intensity will shift from the biceps to the lats. At this level and beyond, the elbow will experience a lot more stress in the overhand grip. For that reason, it is better to use only the underhand grip.

Advanced
Progressions

One-Arm Eye-Level Bent Arm Hang

Muscles Worked

Front: Pectorals, Front Deltoids, Biceps, Grip Muscles, Abdominals, Obliques, Serratus

Back: Rear Deltoids, Rotator Cuff, Trapezius, Lats, Rhomboids

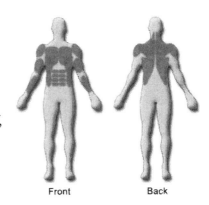

Front   Back

One-Arm Pull-Up Hang

Difficulty: ★★★★★

Directions

From a one-arm dead hang on the bar, pull your body up and hold when the bar is just below your chin.

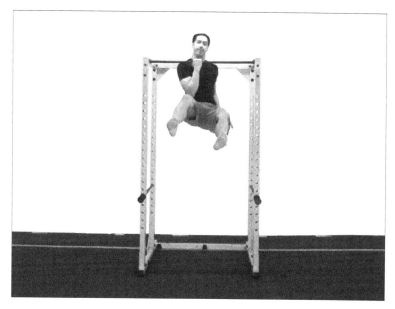

Comments

You should be engaging your lats and upper back muscles very intensely at this point. At this level and beyond, the elbow will experience a lot more stress in the overhand grip. For that reason, it is better to use only the underhand grip.

Advanced
Progressions

One-Arm Pull-Up Hang

Muscles Worked

Front: Pectorals, Front Deltoids, Biceps, Grip Muscles, Abdominals, Obliques, Serratus

Back: Rear Deltoids, Rotator Cuff, Trapezius, Lats, Rhomboids

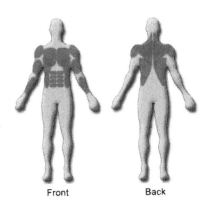

Front   Back

One-Arm Super Pull-Up Hang

Difficulty: ★★★★★ +

Directions

From a one-arm dead hang on the bar, pull your body up and hold when the bar is at the level of your upper chest.

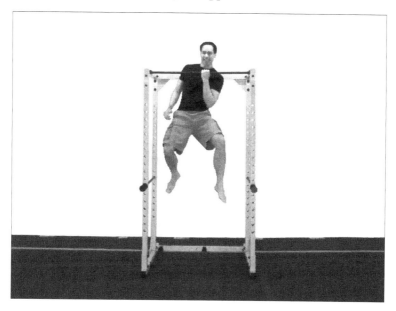

Comments

This is an extremely difficult exercise and it starts working on the one-armed pushing movement. There can be a lot of strain on your muscles, tendons, and joints. If you feel pain when doing this exercise, stop immediately to prevent injury. With time, your muscles and joints will get stronger, but if you push them too fast, they will get injured. Injury will require rest to recover, which will push your progress back significantly. It is better to take it slow than to get injured. At this level, the elbow will experience a lot more stress in the overhand grip. For that reason, it is better to use only the underhand grip.

Advanced
Progressions

One-Arm Super Pull-Up Hang

Muscles Worked

Front: Pectorals, Biceps, Grip Muscles, Abdominals, Obliques, Serratus

Back: Rear Deltoids, Rotator Cuff, Triceps, Trapezius, Lats, Rhomboids

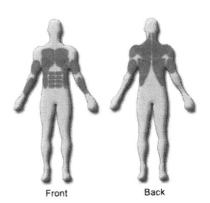

Front   Back

33

Iron Crosses

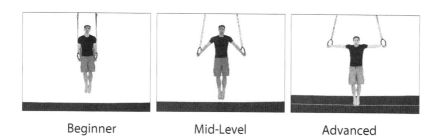

| Beginner | Mid-Level | Advanced |

The Iron Cross is an impressive display of strength that is quite difficult to achieve. Not only do all of the muscles in the upper body need to be strong enough, the joints and tendons need to be prepared for this intense exercise as well. Progressions are a great way to work toward the Iron Cross because of the incremental loading as you go through the exercises. Each exercise prepares your muscles, joints and tendons for the next one until you finally reach the full Iron Cross.

Aside from pure strength, there are technique-related details that are important to remember when training to do the full Iron Cross. Shoulder and elbow position are the first details that you will encounter during your training. Both joints need to be stabilized in order for you to exert the massive amounts of strength necessary to perform this move.

To stabilize your shoulder joint, roll your shoulders forward and squeeze your shoulder blades together. Pull down on your shoulders so that they are pulled down into their sockets. To stabilize your elbows, rotate them so that the elbow pit faces toward the ground. Your biceps will get an intense workout as they work to keep your elbow from hyperextending while in this position. Using this technique will enable you to move on to more advanced positions, such as a Maltese Cross (to be covered in another book). Also, it positions your arms so that you can transition smoothly to more elevated positions. This means you will be able to move upward into different positions, such as the planche and press handstands.

You can use a false grip or a regular grip on the rings for the Iron Cross. A false grip will be easier because you will be supporting your body on your wrists, which are closer to your shoulders than your palms. This reduces the amount of leverage your muscles will have to work against. As you progress in your training, you can also vary the amount of false grip you use. Eventually, you can work out of the false grip into a regular grip, if desired.

The length of your ring straps or cables also makes a difference in the difficulty of this progression. The shorter the supporting straps, the easier the exercises will be, since the rings will be more stable. Shorter straps also help pull the rings together more as you get closer to the full Iron Cross position. So, don't be surprised if you can't hold as difficult a position on rings with longer straps. Once you master the exercises on shorter straps, you can work up to doing them on longer straps.

When setting up your rings, there is no need to place them high off the ground. They just need to be high enough that your feet don't touch the ground when you are in any of the exercise positions. With lower rings, you should be able to hop up into the starting support position instead of expending energy climbing up. When performing these exercises, you can bend your knees to give your feet more clearance. Alternatively, you can tuck them, or even hold your legs out front in an L-Sit position. Note that these variations may be slightly harder, since you will need to engage more muscles. They will also change the balance point, which can target your muscles differently.

Equipment Needed

Exercise rings, gymnastics rings, or similar suspension trainers and a suitable location to use them

Advanced Progressions

Exercise Map

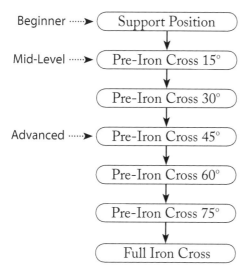

Beginner ·····► Support Position

Mid-Level ·····► Pre-Iron Cross 15°

Pre-Iron Cross 30°

Advanced ·····► Pre-Iron Cross 45°

Pre-Iron Cross 60°

Pre-Iron Cross 75°

Full Iron Cross

Advanced
Progressions

Support Position

Difficulty: ★★☆☆☆

Directions

Get on the rings with your arms straight and hands by your hips, preferably with the rings turned forward and out.

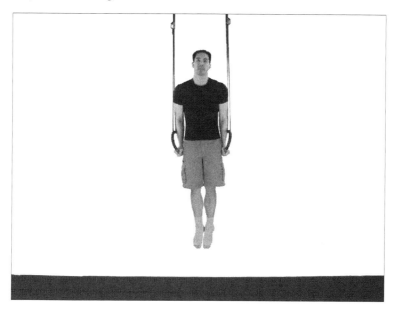

Comments

This exercise is a fundamental skill in ring work. Developing enough strength and control to be comfortable in the support position is a prerequisite for all other supporting ring skills. Turning the rings forward and out will be a little harder at first, but it makes advanced moves easier to do in the future. It is a good habit to establish.

Tips

>> Make sure you push your shoulders down away from your ears so that you can stabilize your shoulders.

>> When you get up on the rings the first few times, you will feel very unstable. The rings will feel like they want to go all over the

Advanced
Progressions

place. Stabilize them by squeezing your arms against your sides. As you get stronger and develop more control, you can move your arms away from your sides.

Muscles Worked

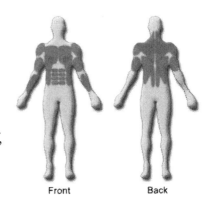

Front: Pectorals, Front Deltoids, Biceps, Grip Muscles, Wrist Flexors, Abdominals, Obliques, Serratus

Back: Rear Deltoids, Rotator Cuff, Triceps, Trapezius, Lats, Rhomboids, Lower Back

Front   Back

Pre-Iron Cross 15°

Difficulty: ★★☆☆☆

Directions

From the support position, move your arms out to the sides until each arm is about 15 degrees from vertical.

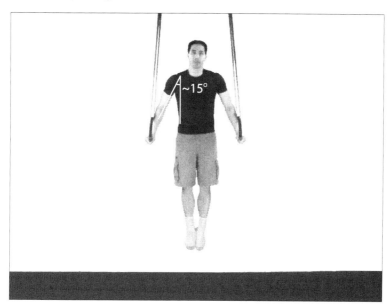

Comments

This exercise starts moving your arms away from your body. Focus on locking out your form and maintaining stability. You may start to feel some load on your biceps, since they will be working to keep your elbow from hyperextending.

Tips

» Keep your shoulders pulled down into their sockets at all times.

» It is a good habit to squeeze your legs together. It is easier to move your legs apart when you are already able to keep them together. It doesn't work the other way around.

Pre-Iron Cross 15°

Muscles Worked

Front: Pectorals, Front Deltoids, Biceps, Grip Muscles, Wrist Flexors, Abdominals, Obliques, Serratus

Back: Rear Deltoids, Rotator Cuff, Triceps, Trapezius, Lats, Rhomboids, Lower Back

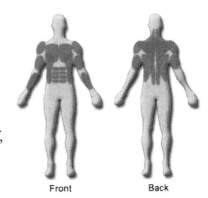

Front   Back

Pre-Iron Cross 30°

Difficulty: ★★⯪☆☆

Directions

From the support position, move your arms out to the sides until each arm is about 30 degrees from vertical.

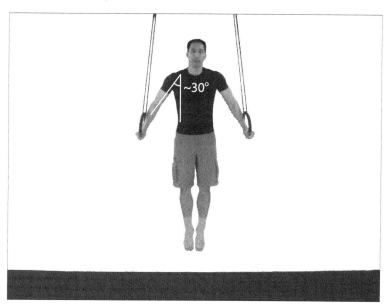

Comments

You should feel an increased load on your arms and upper body in this position. Again, focus on locking out your form and maintaining stability.

Tips

>> Keep your shoulders pulled down into their sockets at all times.

>> Don't forget to keep your legs squeezed together.

Advanced Progressions

Pre-Iron Cross 30°

Muscles Worked

Front: Pectorals, Front Deltoids, Biceps, Grip Muscles, Wrist Flexors, Abdominals, Obliques, Serratus

Back: Rear Deltoids, Rotator Cuff, Triceps, Trapezius, Lats, Rhomboids, Lower Back

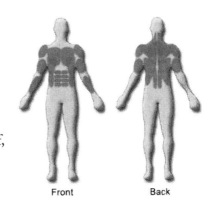

Front   Back

Pre-Iron Cross 45°

Difficulty: ★★★☆☆

Directions

From the support position, move your arms out to the sides until each arm is about 45 degrees from vertical.

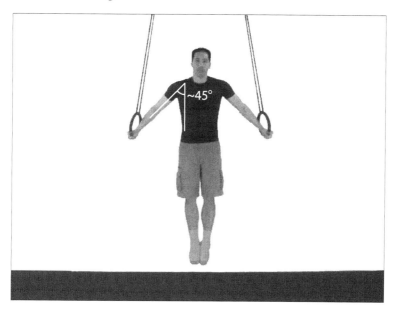

Comments

In this exercise, you are halfway to the Iron Cross visually, although not in terms of difficulty. As you get closer to the full Iron Cross position, the difficulty goes up more quickly for the same increment in arm position. Focus on locking out your form and maintaining stability.

Tips

» Keep your shoulders pulled down into their sockets at all times.

» Don't forget to keep your legs squeezed together.

Pre-Iron Cross 45°

Muscles Worked

Front: Pectorals, Front Deltoids, Biceps, Grip Muscles, Wrist Flexors, Abdominals, Obliques, Serratus

Back: Rear Deltoids, Rotator Cuff, Triceps, Trapezius, Lats, Rhomboids, Lower Back

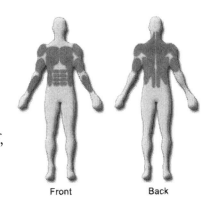

Front   Back

Pre-Iron Cross 60°

Difficulty: ★★★★☆

Directions

From the support position, move your arms out to the sides until each arm is about 60 degrees from vertical.

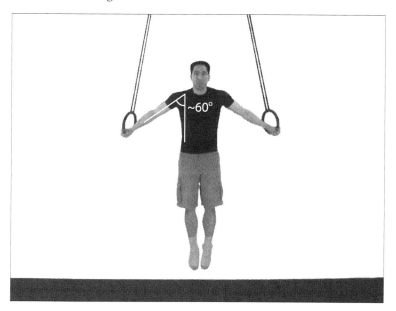

Comments

Now you are getting closer to the Iron Cross. You should be contracting all of the target muscles intensely in order to lock out your form. Remember to keep your elbows straight.

Tips

» Don't forget to breathe! Take shallow breaths if it is difficult to take regular breaths.

» Keep your shoulders pulled down into their sockets at all times.

» Don't forget to keep your legs squeezed together.

Pre-Iron Cross 60°

Muscles Worked

Front: Pectorals, Front Deltoids, Biceps, Grip Muscles, Wrist Flexors, Abdominals, Obliques, Serratus

Back: Rear Deltoids, Rotator Cuff, Triceps, Trapezius, Lats, Rhomboids, Lower Back

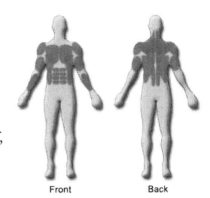

Front   Back

Pre-Iron Cross 75°

Difficulty: ★★★★★

Directions

From the support position, move your arms out to the sides until each arm is about 75 degrees from vertical.

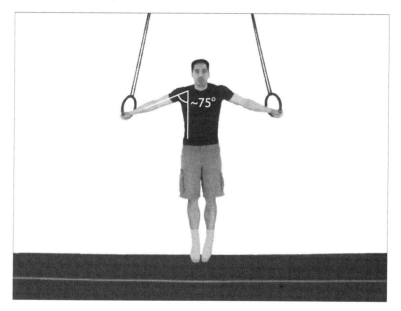

Comments

Almost there! Continue focusing on locking out your form and keeping your elbows straight.

Tips

» Don't forget to breathe! Take shallow breaths if it is difficult to take regular breaths.

» Keep your shoulders pulled down into their sockets at all times.

» Don't forget to keep your legs squeezed together.

Advanced
Progressions

Pre-Iron Cross 75°

Muscles Worked

Front: Pectorals, Front Deltoids, Biceps, Grip Muscles, Wrist Flexors, Abdominals, Obliques, Serratus

Back: Rear Deltoids, Rotator Cuff, Triceps, Trapezius, Lats, Rhomboids, Lower Back

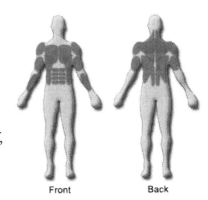

Front   Back

Full Iron Cross

Difficulty: ★★★★★ **+**

Directions

From the support position, move your arms out to the sides until they are fully horizontal and parallel to the floor.

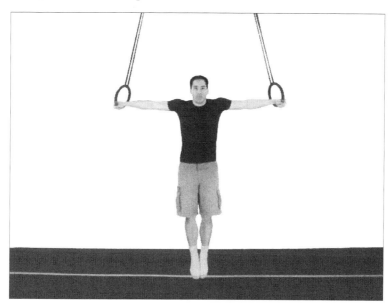

Comments

You're finally there! This is the full Iron Cross. As in all of the previous exercises, focus on locking out your form and keeping your elbows straight.

Tips

» Don't forget to breathe! Take shallow breaths if it is difficult to take regular breaths.

» Keep your shoulders pulled down into their sockets at all times.

» Don't forget to keep your legs squeezed together.

**Advanced
Progressions**

Full Iron Cross

Muscles Worked

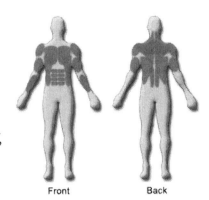

Front: Pectorals, Front Deltoids, Biceps, Grip Muscles, Wrist Flexors, Abdominals, Obliques, Serratus

Back: Rear Deltoids, Rotator Cuff, Triceps, Trapezius, Lats, Rhomboids, Lower Back

Front   Back

34

Flags

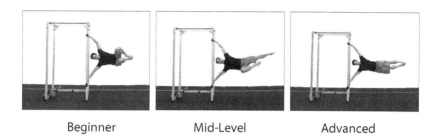

Beginner   Mid-Level   Advanced

The Flag Progression is a great way to build exceptional side core strength as well as arm and shoulder strength. These exercises require a good amount of balance, as it is easy to sway to the front or back and lose your form. The key is maintaining a tight core and establishing a strong, locked-out support from the bottom arm and shoulder. You may find it easier to bend the upper arm, since this will change your body angle and reduce the load on your core. Eventually, you should work on straightening out the upper arm so that your upper body is horizontal.

When getting into the flag position, first position your hands at the desired points on the support. It is easier with your arms farther apart. Play around with the distance between your arms until you find one that feels comfortable to you. Once you have your hand positions figured out, lock out the bottom arm and shoulder.

If you are working on a set of horizontal bars, grab the lower bar with your palm facing up. It will be easier to support yourself with this grip. Grip the top bar with whichever grip feels natural to you.

If you are working on a vertical pole, grab the pole with the thumb of your bottom hand pointing down and bottom elbow pit pointing up.

This will make it easier to establish a solid bottom support. The top hand can grip the pole with either an overhand or underhand grip. I personally find it easier to use an underhand grip, since it enables me to balance myself better.

Next, you will need to get your legs into position. One method is to jump up so your legs are in position at the top of the jump. Another method is to pull both legs up into position at the same time. Yet another alternative is holding the top leg up in the desired position, then pulling the lower leg into position. This is generally the easiest, since your legs move into position gradually. This reduces the risk of your legs swinging down after a jump or double-leg pull.

While this exercise works intensely on the side core muscles, you will need to engage your front and back core muscles to maintain your balance. Otherwise, your hips will start twisting and pull you off of the support. Finally, since this is a one-sided progression, be sure to work the other side equally.

Equipment Needed

A vertical pole, stall bars, or similar stable setup capable of supporting several times your weight

Exercise Map

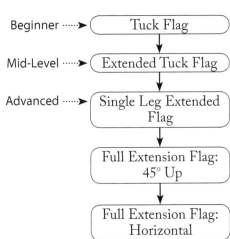

Tuck Flag

Difficulty: ★★☆☆☆

Directions

Position your hands on the support, then enter the flag position, keeping your body tucked.

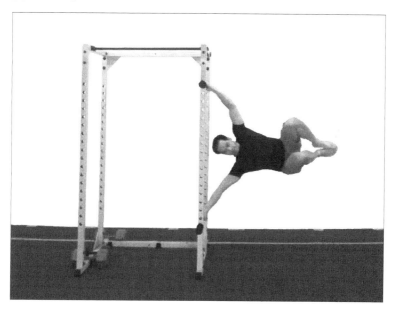

Comments

This exercise gives you a feel for the flag position. Focus on pressing down with your bottom arm and shoulder so that it provides a solid support.

Tips

» Pull up with your upper arm, bending it a bit if necessary.

» Try to maintain a tight tuck, but do not bring your knees up to your chest. Doing so will throw you off balance. Instead, bring your feet close to your butt with your knees somewhat in front. As you get stronger and more familiar with the flag position, your balance will improve.

Advanced
Progressions

Tuck Flag

Muscles Worked

Front: Pectorals, Front Deltoids, Biceps, Grip Muscles, Abdominals, Obliques, Serratus

Back: Rear Deltoids, Rotator Cuff, Triceps, Trapezius, Lats, Rhomboids, Lower Back

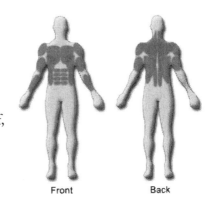

Front   Back

Extended Tuck Flag

Difficulty: ★★☆☆☆

Directions

Position your hands on the support, then enter the flag position, keeping your body in an extended tuck.

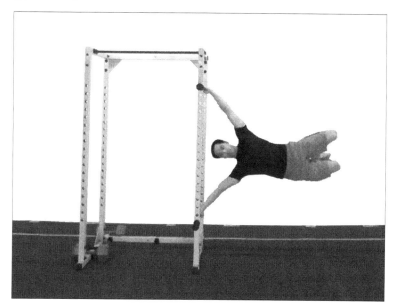

Comments

This exercise is similar to the previous exercise, but the extended tuck increases the load on your target muscles.

Tips

» Focus on keeping your core engaged so that you can maintain your balance.

» Do not let your legs go too far behind you, or you will be pulled off of the support.

Extended Tuck Flag

Muscles Worked

Front: Pectorals, Front Deltoids, Biceps, Grip Muscles, Abdominals, Obliques, Serratus, Hip Flexors, Hip Adductors

Back: Rear Deltoids, Rotator Cuff, Triceps, Trapezius, Lats, Rhomboids, Lower Back, Gluteus Maximus, Hip Abductors

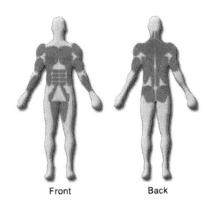

Front   Back

Single Leg Extended Flag

Difficulty: ★★★☆☆

Directions

Position your hands on the support, then enter the flag position, keeping one leg tucked and the other fully extended.

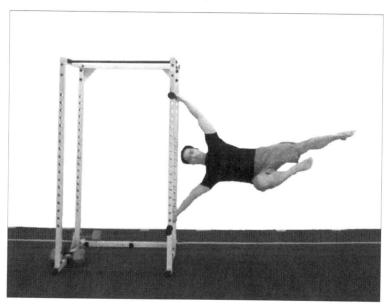

Comments

Extending one leg increases the load on the target muscles even more.

Tips

» It is generally easier to extend the top leg first.

» If you find this difficult, you can raise the extended leg upward at an angle to reduce the load. This will help you develop the strength necessary to maintain the single leg extended position. Eventually, you will want to work the extended leg into a fully horizontal position.

Single Leg Extended Flag

Muscles Worked

Front: Pectorals, Front Deltoids, Biceps, Grip Muscles, Abdominals, Obliques, Serratus, Hip Flexors, Hip Adductors, Quads

Back: Rear Deltoids, Rotator Cuff, Triceps, Trapezius, Lats, Rhomboids, Lower Back, Gluteus Maximus, Hip Abductors, Hamstrings

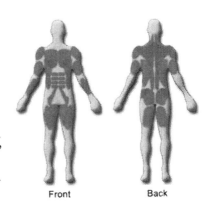

Front   Back

Full Extension Flag: 45° Up

Difficulty: ★★★✬☆

Directions

Position your hands on the support, then enter the flag position, keeping your body and both legs fully extended and pointing upward at a 45-degree angle.

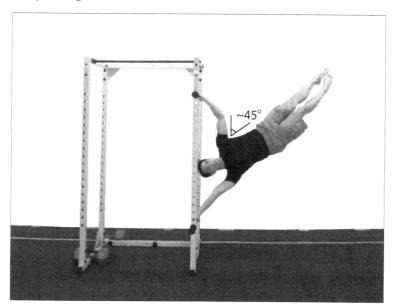

Comments

This exercise approaches the fully horizontal extended flag, but makes it easier by angling the legs upward. Remember to focus on keeping the bottom arm fully extended and locked out so you have a good support to work with.

Tips

» If needed, you can bend your top elbow a bit. However, as you get stronger, you will want to work on this exercise with a straight top arm.

Full Extension Flag: 45° Up

Muscles Worked

Front: Pectorals, Front Deltoids, Biceps, Grip Muscles, Abdominals, Obliques, Serratus, Hip Flexors, Hip Adductors, Quads

Back: Rear Deltoids, Rotator Cuff, Triceps, Trapezius, Lats, Rhomboids, Lower Back, Gluteus Maximus, Hip Abductors, Hamstrings

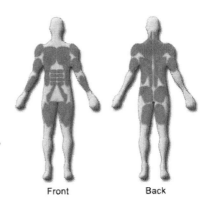

Front   Back

Full Extension Flag: Horizontal

Difficulty: ★★★★⯪

Directions

Position your hands on the support, then enter the flag position, keeping your body and both legs fully extended and horizontal.

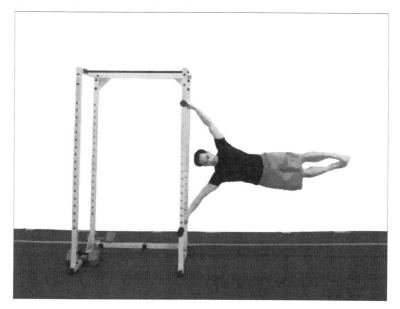

Comments

This exercise is the full horizontal flag. The key is to have strong stable support from the bottom arm and a tight core. Once you get into position, you'll need to focus on maintaining your balance so you do not fall off.

Tips

» If needed, you can bend your top elbow a bit. However, as you get stronger, you will want to work on this exercise with a straight top arm.

Full Extension Flag: Horizontal

Muscles Worked

Front: Pectorals, Front Deltoids, Biceps, Grip Muscles, Abdominals, Obliques, Serratus, Hip Flexors, Hip Adductors, Quads

Back: Rear Deltoids, Rotator Cuff, Triceps, Trapezius, Lats, Rhomboids, Lower Back, Gluteus Maximus, Hip Abductors, Hamstrings

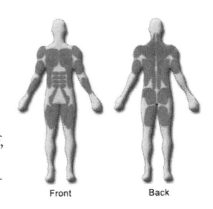

Front   Back

Appendix

One Minute Workout Tracker

The following pages contain copies of the One Minute Workout paper tracker. You can use these to log your exercise sessions. Look back at your progress periodically and you'll be amazed at what you have accomplished. The satisfaction you get from making progress will help you stay motivated.

If you prefer tracking your workouts electronically, visit the One Minute Workout website at www.OneMinWorkout.com. When you sign up for the online virtual trainer service, it will keep track of your exercise sessions and suggest what exercises to do each day based on your goals and workout history. You can also opt to have customized workout reminders sent to you throughout the day. This way, you don't even have to think about what to do, or when to work out. Finally, there is also a convenient voice counter that you can use to time your workouts. This service is what I personally use to keep myself on track.

My One Minute Workouts

Date	Progression	Exercise	Seconds				
8/1/2014	Front Plank	Arms Forward Lv 1	15	10	10	10	5
			5	5			

Need more space? Download printable copies from www.OneMinWorkout.com.

My One Minute Workouts

Date	Progression	Exercise	Seconds				

Need more space? Download printable copies from www.OneMinWorkout.com.

One Minute Workout Programs

Below, you'll find some sample workout programs that you can follow. Once you reach the end of a program, just go back to the beginning. These are just examples so feel free to change things around to find what works best for you!

OMW Minimum Basics

Monday	Tuesday	Wednesday	Thursday	Friday	Saturday	Sunday
Sit Press	Squat	Front Plank	Sit Press	Squat	Front Plank	Rest

Note: As the name suggests, this is a bare-bones program that covers only the most fundamental Basic Progressions. While it can help build a good foundation of strength, I recommend using the OMW Essential Basics Program for better all-around strength.

OMW Essential Basics

Monday	Tuesday	Wednesday	Thursday	Friday	Saturday	Sunday
Sit Press	Squat	Front Plank	Front Leg Raise	Back Plank	Rest	Rest

Note: This program contains two Rest days. If you want to progress more quickly, you can take out one of the Rest days and make it a 6-day program. Alternatively, you can add another progression to the program and do it on one of the Rest days.

OMW All Basics

Monday	Tuesday	Wednesday	Thursday	Friday	Saturday	Sunday
Sit Press	Squat	Front Plank	Side Leg Raise	Back Plank	Front Leg Raise	Rest
Monday	**Tuesday**	**Wednesday**	**Thursday**	**Friday**	**Saturday**	**Sunday**
Side Plank	Back Leg Raise	Back Lean Leg Raise	Sit Press	Squat	Front Plank	Rest
Monday	**Tuesday**	**Wednesday**	**Thursday**	**Friday**	**Saturday**	**Sunday**
Side Leg Raise	Back Plank	Front Leg Raise	Side Plank	Back Leg Raise	Back Lean Leg Raise	Rest

OMW All Basics & Advanced

Monday	Tuesday	Wednesday	Thursday	Friday	Saturday	Sunday
Sit Press	Squat	Front Plank	Hand-Stand	Side Leg Raise	Planche	Rest

Monday	Tuesday	Wednesday	Thursday	Friday	Saturday	Sunday
Back Lever	Back Leg Raise	Pull-Up	Front Leg Raise	Back Plank	Front Lever	Rest

Monday	Tuesday	Wednesday	Thursday	Friday	Saturday	Sunday
Iron Cross	Back Lean Leg Raise	Side Plank	Flag	One Arm Pull-Up	Rest	Rest

Note: This program includes all of the Basic and Advanced Progressions. If you want to accelerate progress, reduce the number of days it takes to go through the entire program. You can achieve this by doing more than one progression on some days, or you can replace some of the "easier" Basic Progressions with similar Advanced Progressions. For example, you can switch out the Front Planks for the Planches.

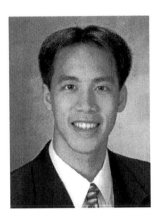

Raymond Wu, M.D. graduated from the Feinberg School of Medicine at Northwestern University and then completed his residency training in Internal Medicine at the McGaw Medical Center of Northwestern University. He has been actively involved in sports for most of his life. Ray holds a black belt in Tae Kwon Do, was nationally ranked in Chinese Wushu Kung Fu, and played college volleyball. Currently, he enjoys biking, tennis, swimming, hiking, ice skating, and gymnastics. Ray's Kung Fu moves can be found in the video game *Mortal Kombat vs. DC Universe*, where he provided motion capture for several characters, and also in his first book, *Fundamentals of High Performance Wushu: Taolu Jumps and Spins*. Besides his passion for playing sports, Ray is an avid computer programmer and founded Transcension Healthcare LLC, a company that specializes in medical simulation software. Originally a New Jersey native, he spent many years in Chicago and currently resides with his wife in Milwaukee, WI.

Printed in Great Britain
by Amazon

35048003R00255